Lisa Annabel Weber

In vitro and *in vivo* development of a topical drug for the treatment of equine skin cancer – based on naturally occurring and synthetically modified substances in plane bark

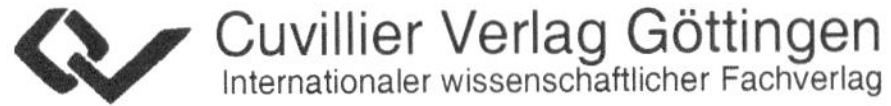

Bibliografische Information der Deutschen Nationalbibliothek
Die Deutsche Nationalbibliothek verzeichnet diese Publikation in der Deutschen Nationalbibliografie; detaillierte bibliographische Daten sind im Internet über http://dnb.d-nb.de abrufbar.
1. Aufl. - Göttingen: Cuvillier, 2021
Zugl.: Hannover (TiHo), Univ., Diss., 2020

Nonnenstieg 8, 37075 Göttingen
Telefon: 0551-54724-0
Telefax: 0551-54724-21
www.cuvillier.de

1. Auflage, 2021
Gedruckt auf umweltfreundlichem, säurefreiem Papier aus nachhaltiger Forstwirtschaft.

ISBN 978-3-7369-7432-6
eISBN 978-3-7369-6432-7

University of Veterinary Medicine Hannover

Clinic for Horses

In vitro and *in vivo* development of a topical drug for the treatment of equine skin cancer – based on naturally occurring and synthetically modified substances in plane bark

---

THESIS

Submitted in partial fulfilment of the requirements for the degree

DOCTOR OF PHILOSOPHY

(PhD)

awarded by the University of Veterinary Medicine Hannover

by

Lisa Annabel Weber

born in Idar-Oberstein

Hannover, Germany 2020

Main supervisor:	Prof. Dr. Karsten Feige
Supervision group:	Prof. Dr. Karsten Feige Prof. Dr. Manfred Kietzmann Prof. Dr. Jessika-M.V. Cavalleri
1st evaluation:	**Prof. Dr. Karsten Feige** University of Veterinary Medicine Hannover, Foundation Clinic for Horses Bünteweg 9 30559 Hannover (Germany)
	Prof. Dr. Manfred Kietzmann University of Veterinary Medicine Hannover, Foundation Department of Pharmacology, Toxicology and Pharmacy Bünteweg 17 30559 Hannover (Germany)
	Prof. Dr. Jessika-M.V. Cavalleri University of Veterinary Medicine Vienna University Equine Clinic Veterinärplatz 1 1210 Vienna (Austria)
2nd evaluation:	**Prof. Dr. Wolfgang Bäumer** Free University of Berlin – Department of Veterinary Medicine Institute of Pharmacology and Toxicology Koserstraße 20 14195 Berlin (Germany)
Date of final exam:	26 October 2020
Sponsorship:	Financial support was provided by the Federal Ministry for Economic Affairs and Energy based on a decision by the German Bundestag (Specific grant number: TopiDrugHorse 16KN051526 BMWI)

Parts of this thesis have been previously published or communicated:

<u>Publications in peer-reviewed journals</u>

Weber LA, Meißner J, Delarocque J, Kalbitz J, Feige K, Kietzmann M, Michaelis A, Paschke R, Michael J, Pratscher B, Cavalleri JMV. Betulinic acid shows anticancer activity against equine melanoma cells and permeates isolated equine skin in vitro. *BMC Vet Res* 2020;16(44):1-9. DOI: 10.1186/s12917-020-2262-5

Weber LA, Funtan A, Paschke R, Meißner J, Delarocque J, Kalbitz J, Feige K, Kietzmann M, Cavalleri JMV. In vitro assessment of triterpenoids NVX-207 and betulinyl-bis-sulfamate as a topical treatment for equine skin cancer. *PLoS ONE* 2020;15(11):1-22.
DOI: 10.1371/journal.pone.0241448

Weber LA, Puff C, Kalbitz J, Kietzmann M, Feige K, Bosse K, Rohn K, Cavalleri JMV. Concentration profiles and safety of topically applied betulinic acid and NVX-207 in eight healthy horses – A randomized, blinded, placebo-controlled, crossover pilot study. *J vet Pharmacol Therap* 2020;00:1-11. DOI: 10.1111/JVP.12903

<u>Oral communications at conferences</u>

27th Annual Conference "Internal Medicine and Clinical Laboratory Diagnostics (InnLab)" of the DVG, Feb 1-2, 2019
Munich, Germany
Weber LA, Meißner J, Delarocque J, Michaelis A, Paschke R, Michael J, Feige K, Kietzmann M, Cavalleri JMV
"Antiproliferative and cytotoxic effects of betulinic acid on equine melanoma cells and percutaneous permeation of betulinic acid through equine skin *in vitro*"
Abstract: *Tierarztl Prax Ausg K* 2019;47(01): 66. DOI: 10.1055/s-0039-1678436

31st European Veterinary Dermatology Congress, Sept 26-28, 2019
Liverpool, United Kingdom
Weber LA, Meißner J, Kietzmann M, Delarocque J, Kalbitz J, Feige K, Michaelis A, Paschke R, Cavalleri JMV
"Anticancer effects of betulinic acid derivative NVX-207 on equine melanoma cells and percutaneous permeation through isolated equine skin *in vitro*"
Abstract: *Vet Dermatol* 2019;30(6): 468–469. DOI: 10.1111/vde.12812

12th European College of Equine Internal Medicine Congress, Nov 22-23, 2019
Valencia, Spain
Weber LA, Meißner J, Feige K, Kietzmann M, Kalbitz J, Delarocque J, Michaelis A, Paschke R, Brandt S, Cavalleri JMV
"*In vitro* assessment of betulinic acid derivative NVX-207 as a topical treatment for equine sarcoids"

12th Graduate School Days, Nov 29-30, 2019
Bad Salzdetfurth, Germany
Weber LA, Kalbitz J, Meißner J, Feige K, Kietzmann M, Puff C, Cavalleri JMV
"Betulinic acid derivative NVX-207: *In vitro* and *in vivo* permeation studies on equine skin"

Poster presentations at conferences

11th European College of Equine Internal Medicine Congress, Nov 9-10, 2018
Ghent, Belgium
Weber LA, Meißner J, Delarocque J, Kalbitz J, Feige K, Kietzmann M, Michaelis A, Paschke R., Michael J, Pratscher B, Cavalleri JMV
"Antiproliferative and cytotoxic effects of betulinic acid and derivatives on equine melanoma cells"
Abstract: *J Vet Intern Med* 2019; 33(3):1555–1556. DOI: 10.1111/jvim.15447

11th Graduate School Days, Nov 30-Dec 1, 2018
Hannover, Germany
Weber LA, Meißner J, Delarocque J, Kalbitz J, Feige K, Kietzmann M, Michaelis A, Paschke R, Michael J, Pratscher B, Cavalleri JMV
"Trees against equine skin cancer? - Antiproliferative and cytotoxic effects of betulinic acid and derivatives on equine melanoma cells"

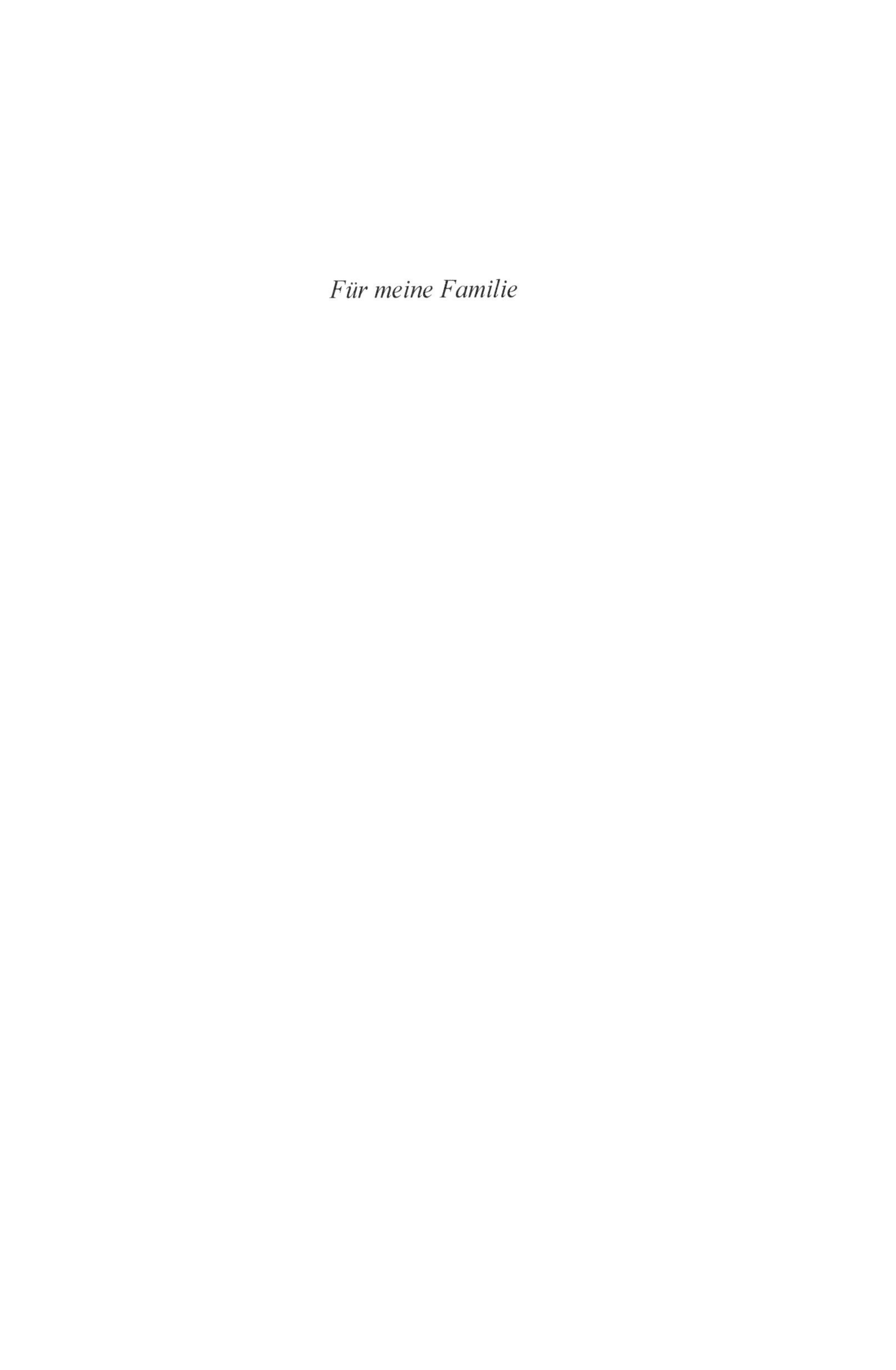

Für meine Familie

TABLE OF CONTENTS

LIST OF ABBREVIATIONS

ASIP	agouti signaling peptide
BA	betulinic acid (3β-hydroxy-lup-20(29)-en-28-oic acid)
BBS	betulinyl-bis-sulfamate ((3β)-Lup-20(29)-ene-3,28-diol, 3,28-disulfamate)
b.i.d.	bis in die = twice a day
BSA	bovine serum albumin
CVS	crystal violet staining assay
DAC	Deutscher Arzneimittel-Codex (German Drug Codex)
DMSO	dimethyl sulfoxide
EMM	equine malignant melanoma
eRGO1	equine melanoma cells Research Group Oncology 1
ES	equine sarcoid
FACS	fluorescence-activated cell sorting
FBS	fetal bovine serum
FDC	Franz-type diffusion cell
HPLC	high-performance liquid chromatography
IC_{50}	half-maximal inhibitory concentration
MelDuWi	(equine) melanoma cells Durán Willenbrock
MTS	CellTiter 96®AQ$_{ueous}$ One Solution Cell Proliferation Assay
MW	molecular weight
NR4A3	nuclear receptor subfamily 4, group A, member 3
NVX-207	3-acetyl-betulinic acid-2-amino-3-hydroxy-2-hydroxy methyl-propanoate
PBS	phosphate-buffered saline
PriFi1 / 2	primary equine dermal fibroblasts 1 / 2
rpm	rounds per minute
RACK1	receptor for activated C kinase 1
sRGO1 / 2	(equine) sarcoid cells Research Group Oncology 1 / 2
STX17	syntaxin 17
TF	test formulation
UV	ultraviolet

SUMMARY

Lisa Annabel Weber

In vitro and _in vivo_ development of a topical drug for the treatment of equine skin cancer – based on naturally occurring and synthetically modified substances in plane bark

Skin cancer is a major area of interest within the field of equine oncology. Equine sarcoids (ES) and equine malignant melanoma (EMM) are among the tumors affecting horses diagnosed most frequently. Both cutaneous neoplasms can be a significant cause of economic losses, morbidity and mortality in the animals, whereby the latter two points explain the necessity for treatment from an ethical and medical point of view. However, despite the sophistication of modern equine medicine, the treatment of equine skin cancer can be challenging and established, evidence-based therapies resulting in sustained tumor regression are rare. The topical treatment approach for skin tumors has many advantages, including the possibility of medicating lesions at localizations difficult to reach, high local drug concentration with few to no systemic side effects and low logistical effort. The pentacyclic, lupane-type triterpenes betulinic acid (BA) and betulin can be isolated from many botanical sources, predominantly from the bark of white birch and plane trees. In addition to various biological properties, they have gained attention mainly due to their anticancer features. Within the framework of the current PhD project, the compounds BA, BA derivative NVX-207, and betulin derivative betulinyl-bis-sulfamate (BBS) were assessed for their potential as an epicutaneous therapy for ES and EMM. This thesis comprises various *in vitro* and *in vivo* studies described in four manuscripts, all with the overall purpose of contributing to the development of a topical drug for the treatment of equine skin cancer.

As detailed in manuscript I and II, the compounds BA, NVX-207, and BBS were demonstrated to exert significant antiproliferative and cytotoxic effects against primary ES cells, primary EMM cells, and primary equine dermal fibroblasts in a time- and dose-dependent manner *in vitro*. Importantly, the active mode of action was apoptosis which was assessed by cell cycle analyses and AnnexinV/propidium iodide staining. In contrast to BBS, no clear selectivity for cancer cells compared to the unaltered dermal fibroblasts could be shown for BA and NVX-207. However, the latter two compounds were revealed to be more effective against ES and EMM cells and, therefore, BA and NVX-207 were used for subsequent Franz-type diffusion cell experiments and studies in the target animal. A stable and homogenous distribution of the substances in the 1 % test formulations with "Basiscreme DAC" (amphiphilic cream as published in the German Drug Codex; supplemented with 20 % medium-chained triglycerides for BA) were given. The compounds penetrated and permeated the epidermis and dermis of isolated equine skin and the amounts of BA and NVX-207 detected by high-performance liquid chromatography exceeded by far the previously determined half-maximal inhibitory concentrations of ES and EMM cells. These results were confirmed by *in vivo* permeation studies in eight healthy horses (manuscript III). In the context of these studies, the local and systemic safety of the BA and NVX-207 applied topically were proven by clinical and histopathological examinations and blood analyses. Finally, the topical application of 1 % BA or 1 % NVX-207 twice a day for 13 consecutive weeks in early stage EMM patients proved to be convenient and safe, as shown by the randomized, placebo-controlled, double-blind *in vivo* efficacy study described in manuscript IV. Even though no complete remission of the tumors could be achieved with the pharmaceutical formulations investigated, a clear tumor response was observed after treatment with both BA and NVX-207. However, the findings of the efficacy study must be regarded as preliminary due to the limited group size (six horses each) and need to be verified in a larger cohort. Modifications of the pharmaceutical formulations may further improve the clinical outcome.

In conclusion, the results generated are promising and support prospective investigations of BA, NVX-207 and BBS in both *in vitro* and *in vivo* models aiming at developing a topical therapy for the treatment of ES and EMM. Further advancement of the investigational medicinal products studied herein could lead to an effective topical and marketable, novel drug which helps to relieve suffering and, consequently, improve the welfare of equine skin cancer patients.

ZUSAMMENFASSUNG

Lisa Annabel Weber

In vitro und _in vivo_ Entwicklung eines topischen Medikamentes für die Behandlung des equinen Hautkrebs – basierend auf natürlich vorkommenden und synthetisch modifizierten Wirkstoffen in Platanenrinde

Im Bereich der Pferdeonkologie sind vor allem tumoröse Erkrankungen der Haut von großer Bedeutung. Equine Sarkoide (ES) und equine maligne Melanome (EMM) gehören zu den häufigsten Tumoren, die bei Pferden diagnostiziert werden. Beide kutane Neoplasien können eine signifikante Ursache für wirtschaftliche Verluste, Morbidität und Mortalität bei den Tieren darstellen, wobei insbesondere die beiden letztgenannten Punkte eine Behandlung aus ethischer und medizinischer Sicht notwendig machen. Trotz des hohen Entwicklungsstandes der modernen Pferdemedizin stellt die Behandlung von equinem Hautkrebs noch immer eine Herausforderung für den/die Pferdetierarzt*ärztin dar und etablierte, evidenzbasierte Therapien mit anhaltender Tumorrückbildung sind selten. Der topische Behandlungsansatz für Hauttumore hat viele Vorteile. Hierzu gehören die Möglichkeit zur Therapie von Läsionen an schwer zugänglichen Lokalisationen, eine hohe lokale Wirkstoffkonzentration mit wenigen bis keinen systemischen Nebenwirkungen sowie ein geringer logistischer Aufwand. Die pentazyklischen Triterpene vom Lupantyp Betulinsäure (BA) und Betulin können aus vielen botanischen Quellen, vorwiegend jedoch aus der Rinde von Weißbirken und Platanen, isoliert werden. Sie zeichnen sich durch eine Vielzahl biologischer Eigenschaften aus, unter denen vor allem die antikanzerogenen Wirkungen hervorzuheben sind. Im Rahmen des hier vorgestellten Promotionsprojektes wurden die Wirkstoffe BA, das BA-Derivat NVX-207 und das Betulinderivat Betulinyl-bis-sulfamat (BBS) auf ihr Potenzial als topisches Medikament für das ES und das EMM hin untersucht. Die PhD-Arbeit umfasst verschiedene *in vitro* und *in vivo* Studien, welche in vier Manuskripten beschrieben werden. Alle Studien haben das übergeordnete Ziel, zu der Entwicklung eines topischen Arzneimittels für die Behandlung von Hautkrebs bei Pferden beizutragen.

Es konnte gezeigt werden, dass die Substanzen BA, NVX-207 und BBS *in vitro* signifikante zeit- und dosisabhängige antiproliferative und zytotoxische Wirkungen gegenüber primären ES Zellen, primären EMM Zellen und primären equinen dermalen Fibroblasten haben (Manuskript I und II). Wie mittels Zellzyklusanalysen und AnnexinV/Propidiumiodid-Färbung dargestellt werden konnte, war der aktive Wirkmechanismus die Apoptose. Im Gegensatz zu BBS konnte für BA und NVX-207 keine klare Selektivität für Krebszellen im Vergleich zu gesunden dermalen Fibroblasten gezeigt werden. Die beiden letztgenannten Wirkstoffe erwiesen sich jedoch als wirksamer gegenüber ES und EMM Zellen als BBS, weshalb BA und NVX-207 für nachfolgende Experimente mit Franz-Diffusionszellen und Studien an der Zieltierart verwendet wurden. Eine stabile und homogene Verteilung der Substanzen in den 1 %igen Testformulierungen mit "Basiscreme DAC" (amphiphile Creme wie im Deutschen Arzneimittelkodex veröffentlicht; ergänzt mit 20 % mittelkettigen Triglyceriden für BA) war gegeben. Die Wirkstoffe zeigten eine gute Penetration und Permeation durch die Epidermis und Dermis isolierter Pferdehaut und die mittels Hochleistungsflüssigkeitschromatographie nachgewiesenen Mengen an BA und NVX-207 überstiegen bei weitem die zuvor berechneten mittleren inhibitorischen Konzentrationen für ES und EMM Zellen. Diese Ergebnisse wurden durch *in vivo* Permeationsstudien an acht gesunden Pferden bestätigt (Manuskript III). Im Rahmen dieser Studien wurde zudem die lokale und systemische Verträglichkeit der topisch applizierten Wirkstoffe durch klinische und histopathologische Untersuchungen sowie Blutanalysen nachgewiesen. Schließlich zeigte die in Manuskript IV beschriebene randomisierte, placebokontrollierte, doppelt verblindete *in vivo* Wirksamkeitsstudie die hohe Praktikabilität und gute Verträglichkeit der topischen Anwendung von 1 % BA bzw. 1 % NVX-207 zweimal täglich über dreizehn aufeinanderfolgende Wochen bei EMM Patienten im Frühstadium. Obwohl mit den untersuchten pharmazeutischen Formulierungen keine vollständige Remission der Tumore erreicht werden konnte, wurde ein deutliches Ansprechen der Neoplasien auf die Behandlung mit BA und NVX-207 beobachtet. Angesichts der pro Testsubstanz auf jeweils sechs Pferde begrenzten Gruppengrößen sind die Ergebnisse der Wirksamkeitsstudie jedoch als vorläufig zu betrachten und müssen anhand einer größeren Patientenkohorte verifiziert werden. Modifikationen in den pharmazeutischen Formulierungen könnten zudem das klinische Ergebnis weiter verbessern.

Insgesamt sind die generierten Ergebnisse des vorliegenden Promotionsprojektes vielversprechend und unterstützen prospektive *in vitro* und *in vivo* Untersuchungen mit BA, NVX-207 und BBS, welche die Entwicklung einer topischen Therapie für die Behandlung von ES und EMM zum Ziel haben. Darüber hinaus könnte eine weitere Optimierung der hier untersuchten Studienmedikation zu einem wirksamen topischen und marktfähigen Arzneimittel führen, welches zur Linderung des Leidens und damit zur Verbesserung des Wohlergehens von equinen Hautkrebspatienten beiträgt.

1. Introduction

Skin cancer is a major area of interest within the field of equine oncology. Indeed, cutaneous neoplasms account for about 50 % of all equine neoplasms, making the skin the organ most frequently affected by tumors in horses [1,2]. Four primary skin tumors are mainly diagnosed in horses: equine sarcoid, squamous cell carcinoma, equine melanoma, and papilloma [2,3]. Skin cancer in horses can cause economic losses for the horse owner due to cosmetic issues, breeding impairment and interference with saddle gear [4,5], but it can also lead to serious illness and death of the animal [6,7]. The latter two points in particular make treatment necessary from a medical and ethical point of view. However, despite the sophistication of modern equine medicine, the treatment of skin cancer is still a challenge for the equine veterinarian. For these reasons, the current thesis contributes to the development of a novel veterinary drug for the topical treatment of equine cutaneous cancer. The main focus of the thesis is on equine melanoma, but experiments were also conducted that may benefit the development of a treatment for equine sarcoid. Natural products play an increasing role in the field of anticancer drug discovery, development, and application [8,9] and so the investigated compounds in this thesis are also either directly isolated from botanical sources or they are synthetically modified derivatives of these compounds. The research project on which the thesis is based was part of a collaboration project between the University of Veterinary Medicine Hannover (Hannover, Germany), the Martin-Luther-University Halle-Wittenberg (Halle, Germany), the University of Veterinary Medicine Vienna (Vienna, Austria), Biosolutions Halle GmbH (Halle, Germany), and Skinomics GmbH (Halle, Germany).

1.1. The equine malignant melanoma

Melanomas are malignant tumors of the pigment building melanocytes [10]. Melanocytes derive from neuroectodermal melanoblasts and are mainly located in the skin, especially within the *stratum basale* of the epidermis and in the outer root sheath of hair follicles [11]. In two database surveys with 236 and 964 equine neoplasms respectively, melanomas were reported to account for 4 % – 6 % of all neoplastic lesions [12,13]. However, most reports on tumor incidence and prevalence in the literature are based on histopathologic confirmation. Since biopsies are rarely used by clinicians to diagnose melanoma in horses, the true occurrence is probably much higher [2]. Although melanomas can occur in horses and mules of any hair color, they are primarily a disease in grey-coated horses. In a study with 296 grey Lipizzaner horses the prevalence of melanoma in the overall population was 50% [14]. Another survey demonstrated that 31% of 264 grey Camargue-type horses suffered from these tumors, while the incidence of melanoma was significantly correlated with age [15]. Indeed, reported prevalences of 67% – 80% in grey-coated horses older than 15 years underline the importance of the disease especially in aging animals [14–16]. There seems to be no sex predisposition for the condition [4,17,18].

1.1.1. *Tumor classification*

Currently, a generally recognized classification system for equine melanocytic tumors of the skin is missing. Based on clinical presentation, histopathology, tendency to malignant transformation, and response to surgical excision, some authors distinguish between four manifestations [4,17,19,20]. Briefly, *melanocytic nevi (benign melanocytoma)* are benign-appearing collections of melanocytes located in the superficial dermis or dermo-epidermal junction. They predominantly occur in young horses of any coat color, mostly in sites others than those described for equine dermal melanoma. Surgical excision is generally curative. The rare *anaplastic malignant melanomas* are composed of extremely pleomorphic, occasionally amelanotic epithelioid cells and are typically encountered in aging (>20 years) non-grey and grey horses. They commonly develop lethal organ metastases. *Dermal melanomas* and *dermal melanomatosis* affect grey horses with distinct predilection sites. Both conditions show a very similar histological appearance, presenting as heavily-pigmented tumor cells in the deep dermis, and are therefore classified based on clinical features. *Dermal melanomas* occur in mature, but not aged grey horses as discrete, solitary masses that are surgically excisable. Multiple, coalescing lesions which are often found in aging grey horses are referred as *dermal melanomatosis*. They show a greater potential for metastasis.

Other authors recommend to generally address melanocytic tumors in horses as malignant neoplasms or neoplasms with malignant potential [7,21,22]. As most melanomas in grey horses undergo a transformation from benign to malignant the term "equine malignant melanoma" (EMM), as proposed by Moore and colleagues in 2013 [21], is used in the following.

1.1.2. *Etiology*

A relationship between the grey coat color and melanoma development in horses was already described at the beginning of the 20th century [16,23]. Even though the etiology of melanomas in horses is still not fully clarified, current data suggest that tumor evolution is associated secondary to genetic mutations in the melanin metabolism molecular pathway. Grey horses are born black, bay or chestnut. Due to an autosomal dominant inheritance they turn to a grey phenotype early in life and show a high incidence for vitiligo-like depigmentation and melanoma [24,25]. Compared with heterozygote horses (G/g genotype), homozygous horses (G/G genotype) show a much faster and completer greying process and suffer from greater prevalence and severity of melanomas [23]. The causative mutation for the grey phenotype is a 4.6-kb intronic duplication in the gene syntaxin 17 (STX17) [23,26]. Further, an overexpression

of the neighboring NR4A3 (nuclear receptor subfamily 4, group A, member 3) gene as well as a loss-of-function mutation of the agouti signaling peptide (ASIP) has been suggested to promote dermal melanocyte proliferation in glabrous skin of grey-coated horses [23].
Melanomas in humans have been strongly related with a high exposure to ultraviolet (UV) light [27]. With respect to the dark skin pigmentation, which grey horses maintain throughout their life and which provides good protection against UV light and with regard to the from UV radiation well protected predilection sites of the tumors (e.g. ventral tail, after, guttural pouch), it seems very unlikely that UV radiation has a significant role in the pathogenesis of melanoma in horses [11,28].

1.1.3. Gross pathology and diagnosis

Corresponding to the age when coat-color starts to turn grey or white, the vast majority of tumors appear around the age of five years [19,21]. Early stages of the disease frequently occur as single, black-pigmented, slow-growing and mostly dermally located firm nodules. Predilection sites are glabrous skin regions like the ventral tail root, anus, perineum, external genitalia and occasionally the lips and eyelids [14,15]. Further, they are found on visceral sites in the head (guttural pouch, parotid salivary gland, larynx) [29,30]. With advanced disease multiple and rapid in volume increasing tumors can arise, which frequently present a coalesced, cobblestone-like pattern [19]. Large tumors often ulcerate through the epidermis and exhibit necrotic centers due to deficits of blood supply [18]. Approximately two-thirds of horses affected by melanoma have tumor metastases at necropsy [7,31]. Metastases to any region of the body can occur secondary either to hematogenous or lymphatic spread [7,17], but reports about primary visceral masses exist [7,32,33]. Most common sites for metastases are the regional lymph nodes, liver, lung, spleen, heart, and major blood vessels [7,34] but spinal cord [35] and muscles [7] can be affected also.
Diagnosis can be set clinically based on the typical gross characteristics and localizations of the lesions in conjunction with the horses' signalment (grey-coated). Fine-needle aspirations or biopsies for cytological and histopathological examinations confirm the clinical diagnosis. However, a histopathological determination of the malignancy potential is not always possible [4]. Immunodetection of the receptor for activated C kinase 1 (RACK1) was proposed as a potential marker for malignancy in equine melanoma cells [36].

1.1.4. Clinical signs in diseased horses

Clinical signs depend on the localization of the lesions, the grade of local invasion and presence of internal metastases. Small EMM may simply be a cosmetic blemish but – if localized on the head – can also become sore and infected secondarily through contact with snaffle or bit [4]. If the anal sphincter, penis and prepuce, or vulva commissure are physically obstructed by larger tumors, dyschezia, dysuria, and difficulty with coitus and parturition may result [4]. As for human melanoma patients, mortality in melanoma-affected horses is principally related to metastatic spread to sites distant from the primary cutaneous tumor [37]. However, defecation problems and resulting colic, caused by large cutaneous tumors in the anal area, can also require the euthanasia of the horse. Metastases of EMM have been reported to cause neurologic deficits like lameness of the pelvic limbs, ataxia, dysphagia and Horner's syndrome, but patients are also presented with unspecific signs like weight loss, colic and exercise-intolerance [7,35,38–40].

With regard to the frequently malignant development, the prognosis for horses suffering from EMM is guarded. The clinical problems often arise because of either misjudgment or incorrect management or irresponsible benign neglect of the lesions [11].

1.1.5. Current treatment options

Because of the potential to grow and progress to malignancy, even early stage EMM should be considered rather precancerous than benign – regardless of histopathological classification and slow-growing nature of the lesions [22]. Consequently, any melanoma in horses should be treated [7,11]. Although various approaches have been introduced, there exists no uniformly satisfactory therapy for the disease. Current locoregional or systemic treatment modalities include (cryo)surgery [11,41,42], cimetidine application [43,44], (electro)chemotherapy [45–47], immunotherapy [48–50] and radiation [51,52]. Nevertheless, these therapies are often inefficient, challenging, not commercially available, or lack sufficient data to be considered established. Although the surgical excision may be curative for solitary tumors [41,42], there are limits for surgical interventions when the tumors involved are already confluent or close to important anatomical structures like nerves, vessels, the anal sphincter, or major organs. The local chemotherapeutic approach with cisplatin has been reported to be effective in some lesions [45–47]. However, as a result of its indiscriminate toxicity to both normal and cancer cells the use of the mutagenic cisplatin is linked to strict safety rules [47,53] and, therefore, the therapy is not offered by many clinics.

Commercially available, validated topical (epicutaneous) treatment options for EMM are currently missing. A report exists about the topical therapy of an EMM lesion with toremifene, a triphenylethylene derivative, which resulted in slight tumor volume reduction [54]. Positive therapeutic effects were observed after topical administration of frankincense oil in five EMM affected horses as described in a PhD thesis [55]. However, results of both studies were never confirmed in further evidence-based large-scale trials.

1.2. The equine sarcoid: an overview

Equine sarcoids (ES) are the most common tumors in horses worldwide [56,57]. From 536 equine (muco)cutaneous neoplasms, ES were diagnosed in 51 % of cases and, therefore, exceeded the sum of all other skin cancer in horses, donkey and mules combined [3]. Skin trauma [58,59] and bovine papillomaviruses type 1 and 2 [60–62] play an important role in the etiopathogenesis, but also a genetic predisposition has been associated with the occurrence of the disease [63,64]. Sarcoids are coat-color and gender independent, semimalignant neoplasms of the cutaneous fibroblasts, capable to metastasize into the local tissue and regional lymph nodes but not into internal organs [59,65]. Based upon their morphological characteristics they can be classified in six types: mild occult or verrucous tumors and more severe nodular, fibroblastic, mixed, and malevolent lesions [59]. Predilection sites include the head, neck, extremities, and ventral abdomen, which often leads to interference with bridle and saddle girth and occasionally cause lameness [57]. Sarcoids can significantly affect the animals' welfare, function, and aesthetics due to tumor localization, size, and number. Therefore, the economic value of sarcoid-affected equids is often substantially impaired [57]. The treatment of these skin tumors can be challenging. Thus, it is not surprising that multiple therapeutic approaches have been described, which can be divided into different categories, such as surgery [66–68], chemotherapy [45,69–72], immunotherapy [73–76], radiotherapy [77–79], photodynamic therapy [80,81], phytotherapy [82,83] and others [84]. Their application depends on tumor type, size, number, duration, localization and previous treatments, experience and facilities of the individual veterinarian, compliance of owner and equine patient, and treatment costs [84]. Unfortunately, resistance to therapy or recurrence in exacerbated forms is frequently observed [6].

1.3. Topical drug application

1.3.1. Why the topical (epicutaneous) approach to treat equine skin cancer?

Given the size of equine patients, the logistical effort as well as the costs for diagnostic processes and treatments can be high [11]. Apart from the financial burden and risks associated with surgical removal of tumors under general anesthesia, the localization of EMM and ES can limit the possibility of surgical intervention or lead to complications in wound healing [30,84]. Furthermore, the systemic treatment of cancer-affected horses with chemotherapeutic agents is restricted mainly by high costs for materials and hospitalization but is also not optimal due to possible systemic side effects on normal cells [11].

The topical (epicutaneous) therapy of skin tumors with anticancer drugs is an interesting alternative to maximize local drug delivery into neoplastic lesions with reduced side effects to normal tissues and simultaneously increased therapeutic benefits [85]. Topical treatments, for example in the form of an ointment or a cream, are non-invasive and can easily be applied even to unfavorable tumor localizations. Additionally, the topical approach provides a treatment opportunity associated with relatively low costs for the horse owner. After instruction by a veterinarian, the horse owner can carry out the treatment without the need for special equipment or facilities, which also significantly reduces the stress factor on the horse. The topical therapy of small EMM lesions would be a better alternative to the common practiced approach of benign neglect, which is often advocated by equine veterinarians and horse owners because of the slow-growing nature of the tumors and the lack of reliable treatment methods for this disease [7,21,22]. Although topical therapies for ES treatment are already utilized, they differ in their efficacy and for some preparations only anecdotal evidence exist [69–71,83,84,86]. Thus, an evidence-based topical therapy, which has been investigated by *in vitro* and *in vivo* experiments from the very beginning, is also needed for this form of skin cancer.

1.3.2. Drug transport across the skin

The major challenge in the development of a topical drug is to transport the anticancer substance to the tumor cells in sufficiently high quantities to kill them. Here, the major barrier to be overcome for topically applied compounds is the outermost avascular layer of the skin: the *stratum corneum*. The *stratum corneum* is composed of dense, functionally dead, and with keratin filaments aggregated corneocytes that are surrounded by a lipid matrix consisting of primarily cholesterol, cholesterol esters, fatty acids, and ceramides [85,87–89]. On the one hand, these structured lipids prevent the body from losing water [90]. On the other hand, they block entry of many topically applied drugs [90] and exogenous substances from the environment. In order to deliver an anticancer substance to a tumor localized in the superficial or deep dermis, the substance must first dissolve homogenously in the transport vehicle (e.g. cream, ointment) [91]. After application to the skin, the compound must release from the pharmaceutical formulation and penetrate the *stratum corneum* either between the lipids of the corneocytes (intercellular route) or through the corneocytes (intracellular route) [87]. Although their contribution to drug transfer is low the skin appendages, particularly hair follicles and sweat glands, are also included in skin permeation [85,87,92]. After the lipid milieu of the *stratum corneum* is passed, the agent has to permeate the hydrophilic viable epidermis to reach the superficial and deep dermis [87,91]. However, because of vascularization of the dermis, blood vessels absorb large amounts of the substance and a subsequent systemic circulation takes place [87,91]. Several techniques exist to overcome physiological as well as tumor-induced skin barriers and to favor drug permeation into deeper skin layers. Strategies include the utilization of chemical penetration enhancers like dimethyl sulfoxide or propylene glycol, the use of nanocarriers, such as liposomes and polymeric and lipid nanoparticles, and the application of physical penetration enhancers like iontophoresis and electroporation [85].

In vitro methods such as Franz-type diffusion cell (FDC) experiments with isolated skin [93] are valuable tools for the development and screening of pharmaceutical formulations as they help to predict the *in vivo* cutaneous penetration and permeation [87,94]. Due to possible interspecies differences in skin structure, it is of great advantage if skin of the target species can be used for *in vitro* experiments [95]. However, the whole complexity of biological systems including metabolism, distribution, and elimination of drugs cannot be reproduced by laboratory trials and *in vivo* data may have to follow the initial evaluations [87,94,95].

1.4. Naturally occurring substances in plane bark and their synthetically modified derivatives

In previous (screening) cell culture experiments, the project partners and the author of the thesis tested naturally occurring substances in plane bark (betulin and betulinic acid) and several of their synthetically modified derivatives in EMM cells [96 and unpublished data]. Based on these experiments and existing literature listed below, it was finally decided that the following compounds would be used within the scope of the PhD project: betulinic acid, betulinic acid derivative NVX-207 and betulin derivative betulinyl-bis-sulfamate (Figure 1).

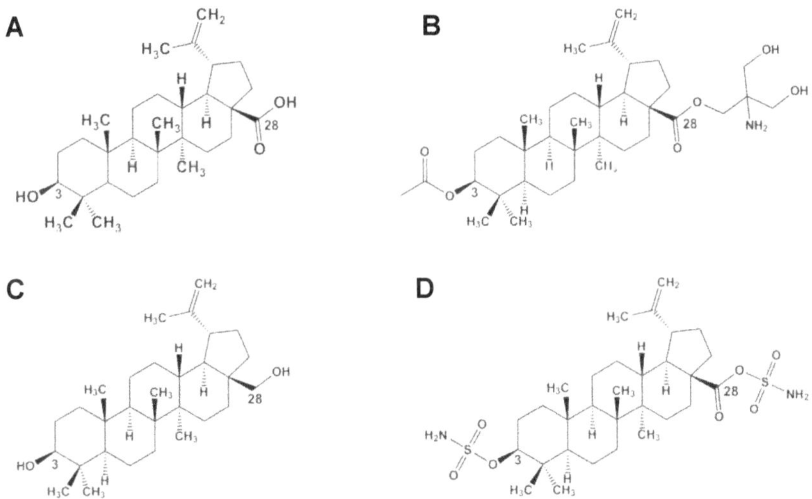

Figure 1. Chemical structures of (**A**) betulinic acid, (**B**) NVX-207, (**C**) betulin, and (**D**) betulinyl-bis-sulfamate.

Structural formulae drawn with ChemDraw (PerkinElmer, Waltham, MA, USA)

1.4.1. Betulinic acid

Betulinic acid (BA; 3β-hydroxy-lup-20(29)-en-28-oic acid; molecular weight (MW): 456.7 g/mol) is a pentacyclic lupane-type triterpene [97]. Triterpene compounds commonly occur in the plant kingdom and perform a protective function against microorganisms and insects [98]. Because of their anti-inflammatory [99–101], antimicrobial [102,103], anthelmintic [104], anti-viral [105,106], and wound-healing properties [107] plants with high content of triterpenes have already been used as phytotherapy in folk medicine since centuries [108]. The compound BA is found in various botanical sources, but considerable amounts can be extracted from the bark of white birch tree species (*Betula* sp.) and plane trees (*Platanus acerifolia*) [109–111]. Furthermore, it can be obtained by chemical or enzymatic oxidation of betulin [110,112]. Since BA's selective cytotoxicity against human melanoma cells was demonstrated in 1995 by *in vitro* cell culture experiments and a murine model [113], a considerable amount of literature has been published on its *in vitro* and *in vivo* anticancer activity against various human malignancies [97,111]. Amongst these are neuroectodermal derived tumors like melanoma, medulloblastoma, glioblastoma and Ewing's sarcoma [115–117], but also ovarian, breast, lung, prostate, renal, and colon carcinoma [114,118]. Many studies reported about BA's mediation of selective cell death in tumor cells, while normal non-cancerous cells of different origin seem to be much more resistant to the compound [113,119,120]. In addition to these *in vitro* observations, the substance was well tolerated in tumor-bearing mice even at high concentrations (up to 500 mg/kg bodyweight) after oral and intraperitoneal application [113,117,121,122]. The antitumor effects of BA are mediated mainly by the activation of the mitochondrial (intrinsic) pathway of apoptosis [115,123]. Through the modulation of pro- and antiapoptotic Bcl-2 family proteins [115,116], BA increases the permeability of the outer mitochondrial membrane [124,125]. Cytochrome *c* and apoptosis-inducing factor are released into the cytosol and the subsequent cleavage of caspases leads to the fragmentation of nuclear DNA and cell shrinkage [123–125]. Additional studies with BA have shown it to induce the generation of reactive oxygen species [115,126,127] which results among others in the activation of proapoptotic mitogen-activated protein kinases [128]. BA-mediated anticancer properties are further explained by the inhibition of topoisomerase I and II [129–131] and induction of antiangiogenic effects within the tumor as a consequence of vascular endothelial growth factor and aminopeptidase N regulation [132–136]. Although extensive research has been carried out on BA's anticancer effects in cells and murine models, no published study exists which reports on the application in human tumor patients. The main disadvantage of BA seems to be its poor water solubility and pharmacokinetic parameters, which limit the use to topical application only [109,110]. Therefore, more than hundred semi-synthetic lupane analogues, derivatives of BA and betulin, were published up to today

[109,110]. For the synthesis of derivatives, modifications of BA and betulin molecules mainly concern active groups at the C-3, C-20 and/or C-28 position [98].

1.4.2. Betulinic acid derivative NVX-207

Amongst a variety of BA derivatives, NVX-207 (3-acetyl-betulinic acid-2-amino-3-hydroxy-2-hydroxy methyl-propanoate; MW: 601.8 g/mol) has been identified as one of the most biologically active and pharmacologically significant substance [96,110,137]. Indeed, NVX-207 shows a higher cytotoxicity in various human and canine cancer cell lines compared to the parent BA [96,137,138]. Besides its more potent activity, significant advantages over BA include a better solubility in aqueous solutions and pharmaceutically suitable solvents [139]. In accordance with BA, NVX-207 was found to induce cell death in cancer cells via activation of the intrinsic apoptotic pathway by cleavage of caspases-9, -3, -7 and poly (ADP-ribose) polymerase [96,137,138], while the impact on the *in vitro* survival of normal human umbilical vein endothelial cells, fibroblasts and keratinocytes was low [137]. An accumulation of EMM cells in the subG1-phase and externalization of phosphatidylserines to the extracellular side of the plasma membrane, a characteristic feature of apoptosis, were observed after treatment with NVX-207 [96]. The compound was already successfully tested in a clinical study with five canine cancer patients suffering from squamous cell carcinoma, soft tissue sarcoma, mammary carcinoma, or adenocarcinoma and clinically beneficial tumor responses including a complete regression were observed [137]. In a pilot safety study with two EMM affected horses the repeated intralesional injection of the compound over 19 consecutive weeks was safe and well tolerated [96]. However, the application of the test substance into the firm tumor tissue required high injection pressures and proved to be difficult, which demonstrates again the advantage of a topical treatment. Summarized, the favorable chemical features of NVX-207 together with the already existing data about its anticancer properties make this substance a well-suited candidate for further preclinical and clinical investigations.

1.4.3. Betulin derivative betulinyl-bis-sulfamate

Betulinyl-bis-sulfamate (BBS; (3β)-Lup-20(29)-ene-3,28-diol, 3,28-disulfamate; MW: 600.3 g/mol) is a derivative of betulin, one of the most commonly found naturally occurring triterpene [98,140]. BBS has been introduced as an efficient inhibitor of human carbonic anhydrase isoenzymes I, II and IX [140]. The cell-surface glycoprotein carbonic anhydrase IX is overexpressed in human melanoma cells and other malignancies [141,142]. It is involved in complex pathways leading to changes in tumor microenvironment (e.g. pericellular acidification) and subsequent tumor progression [141–143]. A combination of proton pump- and carbonic anhydrase IX inhibitors did lead to enhanced anticancer effects in human melanoma cells *in vitro* [141]. Based on these data, BBS could represent a potential candidate as anti-tumor agent alone or as adjunctive therapeutic drug in skin cancer affected horses.

1.5. Hypotheses and aims of the thesis

The overall aim of the thesis was the development of a topical drug for the treatment of equine skin cancer, whereby the main focus of the investigations was on EMM. On the basis of literature and preliminary data, the active ingredient should be based on naturally occurring or synthetically modified substances found in the bark of plane trees. In addition, the compounds were to be tested in ES cells in order to draw conclusions regarding their effects and mechanisms of action and to enforce the generation of new hypotheses for future research projects focusing on the treatment of equine skin cancer. The thesis is organized in four manuscripts either already published in or submitted to peer-reviewed journals. The manuscripts describe *in vitro* and *in vivo* studies that build upon each other and aimed to test the central hypotheses as well as to achieve the overall goal of the thesis.

Hypothesis 1:
Naturally occurring or synthetically modified substances found in the bark of plane trees have antiproliferative and cell viability reducing effects on equine melanoma cells and equine sarcoid cells in vitro. *The mode of action is apoptosis.*

Hypothesis 2:
Naturally occurring or synthetically modified substances found in the bark of plane trees can, when applied topically in an appropriate vehicle, penetrate and permeate horse skin in vitro *and* in vivo *in concentrations sufficiently high enough to exert antitumoral effects against equine skin cancer cells.*

Hypothesis 3:
Topically applied naturally occurring or synthetically modified substances found in the bark of plane trees have antitumoral effects on early stage EMM in vivo.

The **objectives** of the first *in vitro* study, as described in **manuscript I**, were

- to assess the antiproliferative and cell viability reducing effects of BA on primary equine melanoma cells and primary equine dermal fibroblasts
- to demonstrate a selective cytotoxicity of BA to equine melanoma cells, and
- to investigate the penetration and permeation ability of BA in a pharmaceutical test formulation on isolated equine skin

The **objectives** of the second *in vitro* study, as described in **manuscript II**, were

- to investigate BA derivative NVX-207 and betulin derivative BBS for their antiproliferative, cytotoxic and apoptotic effects on equine sarcoid cells, equine melanoma cells and equine dermal fibroblasts
- to assess the more potent derivative for its penetration and permeation on isolated equine skin

The **objectives** of the first *in vivo* study, as described in **manuscript III**, were

- to determine the concentration profiles of BA and NVX-207 in equine skin when applied topically twice a day for seven consecutive days in eight healthy horses
- to evaluate the local and systemic tolerability of both compounds after epicutaneous application.

The **objective** of the second *in vivo* study, as described in **manuscript IV**, was

- to get first insights into the efficacy and safety of BA and NVX-207 in horses with early stage EMM after a 13-week long topical application

2. Manuscript I:

Betulinic acid shows anticancer activity against equine melanoma cells and permeates isolated equine skin *in vitro*

Lisa A. Weber[1†], Jessica Meißner[2†*], Julien Delarocque[1], Jutta Kalbitz[3], Karsten Feige[1], Manfred Kietzmann[2], Anne Michaelis[4], Reinhard Paschke[4], Julia Michael[5], Barbara Pratscher[6,7] and Jessika-M. V. Cavalleri[7]

[1] Clinic for Horses, University of Veterinary Medicine Hannover, Foundation, Bünteweg 9, 30559 Hannover, Germany

[2] Department of Pharmacology, Toxicology and Pharmacy, University of Veterinary Medicine Hannover, Foundation, Bünteweg 17, 30559 Hannover, Germany

[3] Biosolutions Halle GmbH, Weinbergweg 22, 06120 Halle (Saale), Germany

[4] Biozentrum, Martin-Luther-University Halle-Wittenberg, Weinbergweg 22, 06120 Halle (Saale), Germany

[5] Skinomics GmbH, Weinbergweg 23, 06120 Halle (Saale), Germany

[6] University Small Animal Clinic, University of Veterinary Medicine Vienna, Veterinärplatz 1, 1210 Vienna, Austria

[7] University Equine Clinic, University of Veterinary Medicine Vienna, Veterinärplatz 1, 1210 Vienna, Austria

† contributed equally * Corresponding author

BMC Veterinary Research 2020;16(44):1-9

Accepted: 24 January 2020, published online: 05 February 2020

DOI: 10.1186/s12917-020-2262-5

Contribution to the manuscript:

LAW, JM, and JMVC designed the study, analyzed the data and drafted the manuscript. LAW performed cell culture and FDC experiments. JD performed statistical analysis of the data and aided in data analysis. JK developed and performed HPLC analysis. JuM developed the pharmaceutical test formulation. BP aided in cell culture experiments. KF, MK, AM, and RP aided in study design and data analysis. All authors read and approved the final manuscript.

Weber *et al. BMC Veterinary Research* (2020) 16:44
https://doi.org/10.1186/s12917-020-2262-5

BMC Veterinary Research

RESEARCH ARTICLE Open Access

Betulinic acid shows anticancer activity against equine melanoma cells and permeates isolated equine skin in vitro

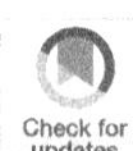

Lisa A. Weber[1†], Jessica Meißner[2*†], Julien Delarocque[1], Jutta Kalbitz[3], Karsten Feige[1], Manfred Kietzmann[2], Anne Michaelis[4], Reinhard Paschke[4], Julia Michael[5], Barbara Pratscher[6,7] and Jessika-M. V. Cavalleri[7]

Abstract

Background: Equine malignant melanoma (EMM) is a frequently occurring dermoepidermal tumor in grey horses. Currently available therapies are either challenging or inefficient. Betulinic acid (BA), a naturally occurring triterpenoid, is a promising compound for cancer treatment. To evaluate the potential of BA as a topical therapy for EMM, its anticancer effects on primary equine melanoma cells and dermal fibroblasts and its percutaneous permeation through isolated equine skin were assessed in vitro.

Results: BA showed antiproliferative and cytotoxic effects on both primary equine melanoma cells and fibroblasts in a time- and dose-dependent manner. The lowest half-maximal inhibitory concentrations were obtained 96 h after the beginning of drug exposure (12.7 μmol/L and 23.6 μmol/L for melanoma cells eRGO1 and MelDuWi, respectively, in cytotoxicity assay). High concentrations of the compound were reached in the required skin layers in vitro.

Conclusion: BA is a promising substance for topical EMM treatment. Further clinical studies in horses are necessary to assess safety and antitumoral effects in vivo.

Keywords: Equine malignant melanoma (EMM), Betulinic acid, Cell culture assay, Franz-type diffusion cell

Background

Betulinic acid (BA), a naturally occurring pentacyclic triterpenoid in the bark of plane and birch trees, has been demonstrated to exert a variety of biological features. In addition to its anti-HIV [1], antiparasitic [2] and anti-inflammatory [3] properties, BA shows anticancer activity in vitro and in vivo [4–10]. Its antitumor effects are mediated mainly by a CD95- and p53-independent induction of apoptosis [11]. Formation of the mitochondrial permeability transition pore complex leads to cytochrome *c* and apoptosis-inducing factor release with subsequent caspases activation [12, 13]. Further molecular antitumoral mechanisms, such as reactive oxygen species formation [14, 15], mitogen-activated protein kinase activation [16], angiogenesis inhibition [17, 18] and other controlled cell death mechanisms [19], have been implicated. Moreover, a selective cytotoxicity on human cancer cells compared to normal cells has been described [5, 20, 21] and might be explained by BA's ability to inhibit the steroyl-CoA-desaturase activity [22]. As tumor cells depend on de novo lipogenesis but not normal cells, inhibition of this enzyme leads to enhanced saturation levels of mitochondrial cardiolipins. Hence, ultrastructural changes in the mitochondrial membrane and subsequent release of cytochrome *c* cause cell death [22]. BA's ability to induce apoptosis has also been demonstrated in equine melanoma cells in vitro [23].

Equine malignant melanoma (EMM) is a common skin neoplasm in aging grey horses [24–26]. An intronic mutation in the STX17 (syntaxin-17) gene was identified as a link to the grey horse phenotype and predisposition to melanoma [27, 28]. EMMs are firm, mostly spherical, occasionally ulcerated tumors of various size arising from the melanocytes mainly in glabrous cutaneous regions [25]. Predilection sites are the ventral surface of

* Correspondence: Jessica.Meissner@tiho-hannover.de
†Lisa A. Weber and Jessica Meißner contributed equally to this work.
2 Department of Pharmacology, Toxicology and Pharmacy, University of Veterinary Medicine Hannover, Foundation, Bünteweg 17, 30559 Hanover, Germany
Full list of author information is available at the end of the article

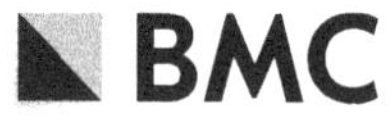

the tail, perineal region, external genitalia, eyelids and lips [29, 30]. Additionally, they are commonly found in the guttural pouch and parotid gland [31]. It has been reported that melanomas represent 3.8% of neoplastic diseases in horses [32]. EMMs progress to malignancy in more than 60% of cases and can cause widespread visceral metastases [31, 33–35]. While some lesions do not cause any clinical problems, others can lead to impaired defecation, colic, weight loss, edema, keratitis and ataxia, depending on the location and size of the tumor [31, 36, 37]. Currently available therapies are either inefficient or challenging. Immunological therapeutic approaches are promising [38] but require further research. Hence, local treatment modalities such as surgical excision, and chemotherapeutic drugs like intralesional cisplatin are commonly used [39–42]. However, unfavorable tumor location might prohibit surgical excision in many cases and the cytotoxic agent cisplatin entails toxic drug exposure risk for the treating veterinarian and any other person coming in contact with the substance (e.g. horse owner, groom) [42]. Thus, more feasible topical treatment options for EMM should be considered. Therefore, the objectives of this study are (1) to assess the antiproliferative and cell viability reducing effects of BA on primary equine melanoma cells and primary equine fibroblasts, (2) to demonstrate a selective cytotoxicity to equine melanoma cells, and (3) to investigate the penetration and permeation ability of BA in a pharmaceutical test formulation on isolated equine skin in vitro.

Results

Cell characterization

Indirect immunocytochemistry was performed to characterize the primary equine dermal fibroblasts. PriFi1 and PriFi2 stained positive for vimentin (Fig. 1), whereas no signal was detected after incubation with anti-cytokeratin. These results, in combination with the spindle-shaped cell morphology, verified PriFi1 and PriFi2 as fibroblasts.

Proliferation inhibition and cytotoxicity of BA on equine cells

The antiproliferative and cytotoxic effects of BA on primary equine melanoma cells and primary equine dermal fibroblasts were investigated. The compound had significant effects on the inhibition of cell proliferation ($P < 0.001$ for CVS for every duration of incubation) and the reduction of cell viability ($P < 0.001$ for MTS for every duration of incubation) on both equine melanoma cells and fibroblasts in a dose-dependent manner. With increasing treatment duration, cell proliferation and cell viability decreased significantly (Fig. 2). A selectivity of the compound to tumor cells compared to normal cells could not be demonstrated (Fig. 2). When cells were exposed to the drug for 5 h, the quantity of cells affected was too low to calculate the IC_{50} values in both cytotoxicity and proliferation assays. The lowest IC_{50} values for all cells were obtained in both, cytotoxicity and proliferation assays, 96 h after the beginning of drug exposure (Table 1).

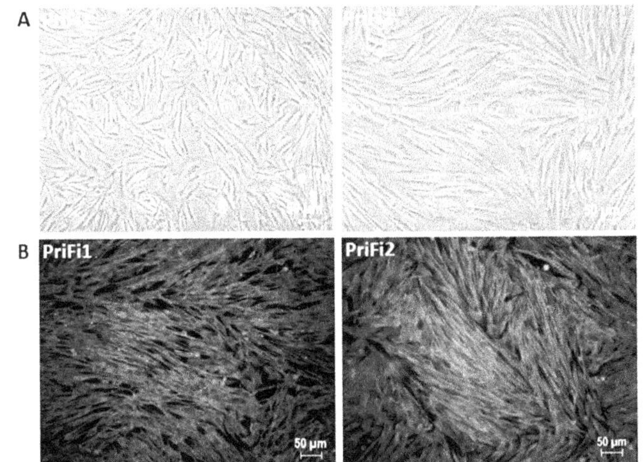

Fig. 1 Verification of dermal fibroblasts (PriFi1 and PriFi2) isolated from the skin of two different horses. **a** Phase contrast microscopy of primary equine dermal fibroblasts PriFi1 and PriFi2. Cells show a typical spindle-shaped morphology. × 10 magnification. **b** Positive fluorescence microscopy detection of intermediate filament vimentin (red fluorescence) in PriFi1 and PriFi2. × 20 magnification, 546 nm

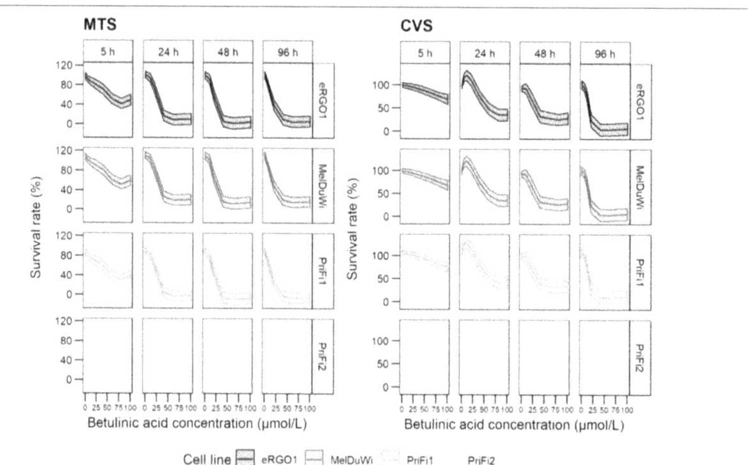

Fig. 2 Predicted mean values and 95% confidence intervals of the survival rates for different equine cells. eRGO1 and MelDuWi = primary equine melanoma cells, PriFi1 and PriFi2 = primary equine dermal fibroblasts. Cytotoxic effects investigated by MTS assay, antiproliferative effects determined by CVS assay. Data represent predicted mean values and 95% confidence intervals of 6–8 independent experiments for each combination of cell type, incubation time and concentration as given by the generalized additive models. BA had a stronger cytotoxic effect when cells were exposed for 24, 48 and 96 h compared to 5 h ($P < 0.001$ each). While there was a highly significant difference in cytotoxicity between 24 h and 96 h ($P < 0.001$), cytotoxic effects differed less between 24 h and 48 h ($P < 0.01$) and 48 h and 96 h ($P < 0.05$). Equally, there was a statistically significant difference in the cell proliferation between a treatment duration of 5 h compared to 24, 48 and 96 h ($P < 0.001$ each). A treatment duration of 24 h compared to 48 h, 24 h compared to 96 h and 48 h compared to 96 h revealed a high significance in cell proliferation ($P < 0.001$ each). A pairwise comparison of all cell types revealed PriFi1 as the most sensitive cell type in MTS assay ($P < 0.001$ for PriFi1 vs. all other cell types), whereas it was the most resistant one in CVS ($P < 0.001$ for PriFi1 vs. all other cell types). MelDuWi was the most resistant cell type towards BA's cytotoxic effects ($P < 0.001$ for MelDuWi vs. all other cell types). In conclusion, betulinic acid did not show a selectivity to equine melanoma cells compared to normal cells

Table 1 IC_{50} values (µmol/L) of betulinic acid for primary equine cells determined by CVS and MTS assay

cells	24 h	48 h	96 h
MTS assay			
eRGO1	22.8 (−3–48)	20.7 (13–29)	12.7 (11–15)
MelDuWi	34.6 (24–45)	31.7 (25–38)	23.6 (13–34)
PriFi1	20.4 (19–22)	18.0 (17–19)	13.8 (7–21)
PriFi2	24.8 (11–39)	22.7 (1–49)	13.3 (11–16)
Crystal violet staining assay			
eRGO1	25.9 (20–32)	21.2 (− 2–44)	19.6 (11–29)
MelDuWi	49.2 (31–67)	35.8 (− 22–94)	21.6 (5–38)
PriFi1	58.0 (52–64)	52.2 (39–65)	14.5 (14–15)
PriFi2	30.3 (17–44)	29.1 (6–53)	13.8 (10–18)

Cytotoxic (MTS assay) and antiproliferative (crystal violet staining assay) effects of betulinic acid on primary equine melanoma cells (eRGO1 and MelDuWi) and primary equine dermal fibroblasts (PriFi1 and PriFi2) after a treatment duration of 24, 48, or 96 h. Data represent mean IC_{50} values (µmol/L) of 6–8 independent experiments with 95% confidence interval in parentheses

Diffusion of BA into equine skin and overall BA recoveries

The penetration and permeation properties of 1% BA with 20% medium-chain triglycerides in "Basiscreme DAC" on isolated equine skin using FDCs were evaluated to identify an effective formulation for prospective in vivo use. An overall BA recovery of 98 ± 7% (mean ± SD; $n = 7$) was achieved. A quantity of 18 ± 11% of the amount of BA applied was detected in the acceptor media and 56 ± 13% in the cotton swabs. In the skin, 24 ± 1% of the BA amount applied was analyzed, from which 9 ± 7% were found in the blade cleaning tissues. BA was able to penetrate the *stratum corneum* and permeate through the epidermal and dermal layers of the isolated equine skin within 24 h (Fig. 3). At a depth of 810 µm, the concentration of BA was still 39.6 µmol/L ± 38 µmol/L (mean ± SD). Including this skin layer, the BA concentration in isolated equine skin exceeded the 24-h IC_{50} values of both equine melanoma cells and fibroblasts investigated by the cytotoxicity assay in all layers examined. Up to a depth of 710 µm, the 24-h IC_{50} values of equine melanoma cells investigated by proliferation assay were surpassed (55.8 µmol/L ± 31 µmol/L).

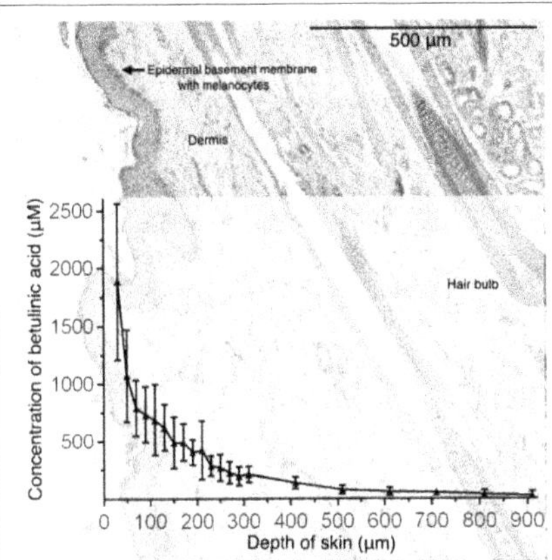

Fig. 3 Concentration profile of betulinic acid correlative to skin thickness. Thoracic skin of seven horses (two technical replicates each) were used for 24-h Franz-type diffusion cell experiments with "Basiscreme DAC" containing 1% betulinic acid and 20% medium-chain triglycerides. Data represent mean concentration (±SD) of betulinic acid in cryostat skin slices at different skin depths. Detected amounts of BA by far exceeded the determined IC_{50} values for equine melanoma cells after 24 h, especially in the uppermost skin layers (410 µm). As minor cream residues on the skin surface after cleaning with a cotton swab cannot be excluded, data for 10 µm skin depth were eliminated in this figure. Hematoxylin and eosin staining of equine lateral thoracic skin kindly provided by the Institute for Anatomy, University of Veterinary Medicine Hannover, Foundation, Hannover, Germany

Discussion

The aim of these in vitro studies was to explore the potential of BA as a topical therapy against EMM. Antiproliferative and cytotoxic effects of the compound on primary equine melanoma cells and primary equine dermal fibroblasts as well as its permeation through isolated equine skin were investigated. It could be shown that BA inhibits proliferation and cell metabolism in equine melanoma cells and dermal fibroblasts in a time- and dose-dependent manner. Moreover, when 1% BA in "Basiscreme DAC" supplemented with 20% medium-chained triglycerides was applied on isolated equine skin, high concentrations of the compound were reached in the required skin layers.

Antiproliferative and cytotoxic effects were observable as early as after 5 h of drug exposition, however, at this time point the quantity of cells affected was too low to calculate IC_{50} values. The results demonstrate that antiproliferative and cytotoxic effects increase with treatment duration and thus the lowest IC_{50} values were obtained 96 h after the beginning of drug exposure. With the four different incubation time points and the resulting IC_{50} values, information about the time-dependent cytotoxic and antiproliferative effects of BA on equine cells were added - not only after 96 h, as reported previously for equine melanoma cells [23], but also after 5, 24 and 48 h. This information may be valuable for the design of treatment regimes in further in vivo studies. Previously reported IC_{50} values of equine melanoma cells determined by the sulforhodamine B assay (33.1 µmol/L (MelDuWi) and 33.4 µmol/L (MelJess)) [23] were higher than the ones investigated in the present study by MTS assay (23.6 µmol/L (MelDuWi) and 12.7 µmol/L (eRGO1)) after the same duration of incubation (96 h) with BA. In the MTS assay a tetrazolium salt is reduced by mitochondrial dehydrogenases to a photometrically measurable formazan product, which quantity reflects the number of living cells in culture [43]. The sulforhodamine B dye binds to protein components of fixed cells and does not distinguish between cells with an active mitochondrial metabolic rate and those without [44]. As BA mainly targets the mitochondrial pathway of apoptosis [45], the MTS assay provides an earlier detection of reduced cell viability and consequently smaller IC_{50} values compared to those formerly reported were calculated. In addition, with the crystal violet staining assay it was demonstrated that the compound is able to not only affect the cell's metabolism, but also to inhibit the proliferation of equine melanoma cells in vitro and therefore potentially stop tumor growth in vivo.

However, the results show that normal equine dermal fibroblasts are also sensitive to BA in the concentrations investigated. These observations are in agreement with previously reported low selectivity indices of BA for normal human dermal fibroblasts [46, 47] and attenuated high glucose-induced proliferation of human cardiac fibroblasts after treatment with BA [48]. But they are in contrast to findings in other human normal cells, such as melanocytes, dermal fibroblasts and peripheral blood lymphocytes, which revealed to be more resistant to a BA treatment than cancer cells [5, 20, 21].

The in vitro cell culture studies reported here did not focus on elucidating the molecular mechanisms behind the BA-induced cell alterations. Nevertheless, it was demonstrated before that BA leads to cell cycle perturbations in equine melanoma cells with an accumulation of cells in the $subG_1$-phase [23]. The same authors did demonstrate a BA-related induction of apoptosis in equine melanoma cells by AnnexinV/Propidium iodide staining and proof of caspases 3-, 8-, and 9 activation [23]. A variety of other molecular pathways are described mainly for human cancer cells [49], but need to be verified for equine cancer cells in prospective experiments. The literature about BA's effects towards normal cells on the molecular level is limited. While inhibition of the steroyl-CoA-desaturase is a possible explanation for BA's selectivity to some human cancer cells compared to the non-transformed human fibroblasts Co18

[22], the mechanisms behind the results shown here is not known and further studies on healthy equine cells treated with BA are needed to understand the effective mode of action.

In a clinical setting the compound needs to reach the melanoma cells in the patient to be effective. While some melanomas are ulcerated, most are covered by epidermal and dermal skin layers [50, 51]. Thus, a topically applied substance needs to penetrate the *stratum corneum*, the major barrier for transdermal drugs, and permeate through the epidermal and dermal strata. It was demonstrated that 1% BA in "Basiscreme DAC" with 20% medium-chain triglycerides fulfilled this requirement in isolated equine thoracic skin in vitro. In the FDC experiments amounts of BA were detected that by far exceeded the determined IC_{50} values for equine melanoma cells after 24 h and therefore melanomas located in the superficial and partly deeper dermal layers (up to 810 μm) could be affected by the compound. Due to practical reasons, a standardized use of nearly glabrous skin from EMM predilection sites (e.g. perineal region, external genitalia, eyelids) was not possible. This should be considered a limitation of this study. Nevertheless, others have shown that hydrocortisone, a lipophilic substance similar to BA, penetrated hairy equine thoracic skin in the same manner as nearly glabrous equine groin skin [52]. Therefore, the penetration profile of BA in equine thoracic skin compared to the skin at predilection sites can be expected to be similar.

In vitro FDC studies can be predictive for in vivo penetration and permeation data, but due to the lack of circulation they cannot provide information about the amount of a compound that is eliminated from the skin by capillary dermal blood vessels [53]. In some EMM an increased vascularization was observed [26, 51], which could lead to a higher and faster elimination of the active compound when topically applied in vivo. On the other hand, BAs' potential to reduce angiogenesis was demonstrated in vitro and in vivo by inhibition of hypoxia-inducible factor 1α and vascular endothelial growth factor and by a negative impact on the normal growth of the capillaries in the chorioallantoic membrane assay [17, 18, 54]. Reducing the vascularization in the tumor could increase the drug concentration in this area. Further, therapeutic strategies aiming at anti-angiogenesis are reported as adjunctive therapies against melanomas in human medicine [55].

Summarizing, the potent percutaneous permeation of BA in normal skin together with its anticancer effects on equine melanoma cells suggest that this substance may exert antitumoral effects in vivo. Even if normal equine skin cells are affected by local BA treatment, inflammatory reactions are suspected to be minor, as a topical treatment of actinic keratoses with betulin, a triterpene comparable to betulinic acid, did not lead to any side effects in 14 human patients [56]. Nevertheless, to gain more insights about the therapeutic potential of BA the safety and efficacy of the compound have to be addressed on healthy and melanoma affected equine skin in vivo.

Conclusion

The anticancer effects of BA on equine melanoma cells together with its potent transepidermal and -dermal permeation into the required skin layers make this compound a potential substance for topical melanoma treatment in horses. A selectivity to cancer cells over normal cells could not be demonstrated. In essence, this study supports the use of BA in further preclinical and clinical trials for topical EMM treatment.

Material and methods

Cells and culture conditions

Self-generated primary equine dermal fibroblasts PriFi1 and PriFi2 and previously isolated primary equine melanoma cells were used for the cell culture experiments. The primary equine melanoma cells MelDuWi belong to the cell culture stock of the Clinic for Horses, University of Veterinary Medicine Hannover, Foundation, Germany, while the primary equine melanoma cells eRGO1 were provided by Dr. Barbara Pratscher, Department for Small Animals and Horses, Vetmeduni Vienna, Austria. PriFi1, PriFi2 and MelDuWi were maintained as monolayers in RPMI1640 cell culture medium with stable glutamine (Biochrom GmbH, Berlin, Germany) supplemented with 15% fetal bovine serum (FBS) superior (Biochrom GmbH) and 1% penicillin and streptomycin (10,000 international units (I.U.)/mL / 10,000 μg/mL, Biochrom GmbH) at 37 °C in a humidified atmosphere with 5% CO_2. Melanoma cells eRGO1 were cultured in Dulbecco's modified Eagle's high glucose w/Glutamax (4.5 g/L) cell culture medium (GIBCO-Invitrogen, Thermofisher, Darmstadt, Germany) supplemented with 10% FBS superior (Biochrom GmbH) and 1% Antibiotic-Antimycotic (100x; GIBCO-Invitrogen), containing penicillin (10,000 units/mL), streptomycin (10, 000 μg/mL) and amphotericin B (25 μg/mL).

Dermal cell isolation

Equine dermal fibroblasts were isolated as described by Mählmann [57], with some modifications. A mare (aged 10 years) and a stallion (aged 9 years) without any apparent dermatological disorders were euthanized for reasons unrelated to this study. Immediately after euthanasia, a lateral neck region caudal to the axis (C2) was prepared in accordance with standard surgical aseptic preparation methods. A piece of skin, about 2.5 × 2.5 × 1 cm, was harvested from each horse utilizing a scalpel and forceps. Subcutaneous tissue was removed and the skin was transferred into a sterile 50-mL centrifuge tube containing 15 mL fibroblast culture medium (RPMI1640 with stable glutamine (Biochrom

GmbH), 20 mM HEPES (Sigma-Aldrich, Steinheim, Germany), 20% FBS superior (Biochrom GmbH), 2% penicillin and streptomycin (10,000 I.U./mL / 10,000 µg/mL, Biochrom), and 1% amphotericin B (250 µg/mL, Biochrom GmbH). After transportation at room temperature to the laboratory, the skin was washed three times in sterile phosphate-buffered saline (PBS, pH 7.4; 1 L contains 0.2 g KCl, 8.0 g NaCl, 0.2 g KH_2PO_4, 1.44 g $Na_2HPO_4 \times 2H_2O$ and deionized water). Subsequently, the skin was refrigerated overnight at 4 °C in a sterile centrifuge tube containing 5 mg/mL dispase I (Gibco Invitrogen) diluted in 15 mL fibroblast culture medium without FBS. After 15 h, an incubation step at 37 °C with 5% CO_2 for 2 h followed. Afterwards, the epidermis was separated from the dermis forceps. Dermal tissue was incubated for 8 h with 1 mg/mL (0.15 U/mL) collagenase A (Roche diagnostics GmbH, Mannheim, Germany) and 2 mg/mL (1.6 U/mL) dispase I (GIBCO-Invitrogen) in 15 ml fibroblast culture medium without FBS at 37 °C with 5% CO_2. Meanwhile, the tube was agitated every 2 h. Subsequently, the sample was centrifuged at 450×g for 10 min. After the supernatant had been discarded, the cell pellet was resuspended in 5 mL fibroblast culture medium and sifted through a 70 µm filter. The cells were finally cultivated as monolayers in 25-cm^2 tissue culture flasks at 37 °C with 5% CO_2. After the first passage, the cells were cultivated in modified culture medium (RPMI1640 with 15% FBS and 1% penicillin and streptomycin).

Verification of equine dermal fibroblasts

Equine dermal fibroblasts (PriFi1 and PriFi2) were verified by indirect immunofluorescence staining applying a modified reported protocol [58], except for the secondary antibody and antibody-dilutions. Briefly, a monoclonal mouse anti-vimentin antibody (Clone V-9, Sigma-Aldrich, dilution 1:200) was used. Samples incubated with a monoclonal mouse anti-cytokeratin antibody (C-11, Invitrogen, Rockford, US, dilution 1:100) and those incubated without primary antibody served as negative controls. F(ab')2 goat anti-mouse IgG-FITC antibody (Bio-Rad Laboratories GmbH, Munich, Germany, dilution 1:200) was used for the visualization of the signals. Cells were evaluated and photographed at 546 nm and a 20 fold magnification with a Leica fluorescence microscope (Leica Microsystems, Wetzlar, Germany) and an AxioCam MRc camera (Zeiss Microscopy GmbH, Jena, Germany).

Evaluation of proliferation and cell toxicity of betulinic acid on equine melanoma cells and equine fibroblasts

Pharmacological compounds

Betulinic acid (BA) was provided by Biosolutions Halle GmbH (Halle/Saale, Germany). Dimethyl sulfoxide (DMSO) (WAK-Chemie Medical GmbH, Steinbach, Germany) was used to achieve a 20 mM stock solution.

Proliferation assays

The inhibitory effect of BA on cell proliferation was evaluated using a modified crystal violet staining (CVS) assay [59]. In brief, cells were seeded into 96-well microtiter plates with a density of 5000 cells/well to avert confluence of the cells during the experimental period. Twenty-four hours later, the cells were treated with serial dilutions of BA dissolved in DMSO and medium at nine different concentrations ranging from 1 to 100 µmol/L. The highest concentration of DMSO solvent was 0.5% in 100 µmol/L, which had neither an impact on the cell proliferation rate nor on the cell survival rate (preliminary experiments and regular controls within the experiments; data not shown). Control cells were only treated with medium. The proportion of treated cells in relation to untreated controls was determined 5, 24, 48 and 96 h after the beginning of the drug exposure. The medium for 96-h experiments was renewed before cell treatment (24 h after inoculation). The medium-compound mix was discarded at the time points mentioned above and cells were fixed with 2% glutaraldehyde (Sigma-Aldrich) in PBS for 20 min. Glutaraldehyde was removed and cells were dyed for 30 min with 0.1% crystal violet (Roth GmbH, Karlsruhe, Germany) in deionized water. After washing with deionized water, the plates were air-dried. Subsequently, crystal violet was solubilized out of the cells by adding 2% Triton X-100 (Sigma-Aldrich, Steinheim, Germany) in deionized water. After 1 h of incubation, absorbance was measured at 570 nm using a 96-well microtiter plate reader (MRX microplate reader, Dynatech Laboratories, El Paso, US). Experiments were performed in six to eight biological replicates with two technical replicates for each combination of cell type, incubation time and pharmacologic compound concentration. The ratios of mean optical density of the duplicate to mean optical density of the associated controls were used for dose-response curves.

Cytotoxicity assays

The cytotoxicity of BA was evaluated using the CellTiter 96® AQ$_{ueous}$ One Solution Cell Proliferation Assay (MTS) (Promega GmbH, Mannheim, Germany). Cells were seeded into 96-well microtiter plates with the appropriate cell densities to achieve confluence after 48 h (MelDuWi 30.000 cells/well; PriFi1, PriFi2, eRGO1 20.000 cells/well). After 48 h, these cells were treated in accordance with the CVS assay. Experiments were stopped at the same time points as the CVS assay. The medium for the 96-h experiments was renewed before treatment. The MTS was applied in accordance with the manufacturer's instructions. After 1 h incubation, the plate absorbance was measured at 490 nm using a 96-well microtiter plate reader (MRX microplate reader, Dynatech Laboratories, El Paso, US). Experiments were performed in six to eight biological replicates with two technical replicates for each combination of pharmacologic compound, cell type, incubation time and concentration.

Diffusion of betulinic acid into equine skin

Skin samples

Skin samples from seven adult horses of different sex (three mares, two geldings, two unknown) and breed (including three Warmbloods, one Icelandic horse and one Welsh Cob pony, two unknown) were harvested at the Institute of Pathology, University of Veterinary Medicine Hannover, Foundation, Hannover, after euthanasia at the Clinic for Horses, University of Veterinary Medicine Hannover, Foundation, Hannover, for reasons unrelated to the present study. The horses' ages ranged from 4 to 24 years, with a median of 13.5 years. Skin from the lateral thorax was dissected and stored at − 20 °C for up to 5 months.

Drug formulation

"Basiscreme DAC" (pharmaceutical amphiphilic formulation as published in the German Drug Codex) with 1% BA and 20% medium-chain triglycerides was provided by Skinomics GmbH, Halle, Germany.

In vitro permeation

In order to investigate the penetration and permeation of 1% BA with 20% medium-chain triglycerides in "Basiscreme DAC" through equine skin, the skin samples were defrosted overnight at room temperature. The coat was clipped to a length of approximately 0.5 mm. The integrity of the skin samples was visually assessed. Skin slices of 800 μm (+/− 110 μm) thickness were obtained with an electrical dermatome (Zimmer, Eschbach, Germany). Franz-type diffusion cells (FDC) (PermeGear, Riegelsville, USA, and Gauer Glas, Püttlingen, Germany) with a diffusion area of 1.77 cm^2 and an acceptor chamber volume of approximately 12 mL were filled with PBS and 1% bovine serum albumin. The acceptor chamber content was constantly stirred with a magnetic stirrer at 500 rpm. Diffusion chambers were maintained at 34 °C to ensure a skin temperature of 32 ± 0.5 °C. Before use, equal hydration of the skin samples was obtained by 30 min immersion in PBS. After gently drying with a paper tissue, 20 mg of the drug formulation was carefully applied to the skin surface (*stratum corneum)* covering the complete diffusion area before mounting the skin pieces onto the FDC. The donor chamber and sampling tube were covered with parafilm.

Terminal procedures and BA quantification

After 24 h, the remaining donor formulation was removed from the skin with a dry cotton swab. Cotton swabs, acceptor medium and exposed areas of the skin samples, which were cut out with a scalpel blade, were stored at − 20 °C until further processing and analysis. In order to determine the amount of BA in different skin layers, frozen skin samples were fixed on tissue freezing medium (Leica Biosystems Nussloch GmbH, Nussloch, Germany) and placed in a cryostat (CryoStar™ NX70 Cryostat, Thermofisher, Darmstadt, Germany). From each skin sample slices were cut horizontally to the epidermis, starting with the *stratum corneum* side uppermost, and stored separately. While the first slice had a thickness of 10 μm the following slices were 20 μm thick. After reaching a skin depth of 310 μm, slices were pooled at 5 × 20 μm until a depth of a maximum of 910 μm was reached. The blade was cleaned with tissues soaked in 70% ethanol (CG Chemikalien, Laatzen, Germany) between each cut. These cleaning tissues and skin samples were stored at − 20 °C until final analysis. An analytic high-performance liquid chromatography method was developed for BA quantification in the different skin layers, acceptor medium and cleaning utensils mentioned previously. Reverse phase analysis was performed using an Agilent 1100 system (Agilent, Waldbronn, Germany) on a Kinetex column (5 μm, C18, 100 Å, 250 × 4.6 mm; Phenomenex, Torrance, US) at 35 °C developing with acetonitrile:water (0.1% HCOOH) 4:1 (v/v) at 2.5 mL/min. The diode array detector was set at 200 nm.

Statistical analysis

Technical duplicates with a coefficient of variation of more than 20% were excluded from the analysis of the cell assays. The pharmacodynamic model 108 of Phoenix® WinNonlin® software (version 8.1, Certara, USA) was used to determine half-maximal inhibitory concentrations (IC_{50} values). Further statistical analysis was performed with R 3.5.1 [60]. A generalized additive model was fitted for both MTS and CVS using the 'mgcv' package [61] to estimate the effects of the BA concentration, cell line and duration of incubation on the ratio of the mean optical density of the duplicates from six to eight replicates to the mean optical density of the associated controls. The effect of concentration was modelled as a smoothed term interacting with the duration of incubation using a thin plate regression spline. The *P*-values were obtained by performing a Wald test for each parameter. Post-hoc comparisons for the cell line and duration of incubation were performed using the 'multcomp' package with single-step adjustment of the P-values [62]. Plots were produced with ggplot2 [63]. Statistical significance was set at $P < 0.05$.

Abbreviations

BA: Betulinic acid; CVS: Crystal violet staining assay; DAC: Deutscher Arzneimittel Codex (German Drug Codex); DMSO: Dimethyl sulfoxide; EMM: Equine malignant melanoma; FBS: Fetal bovine serum; FDC: Franz-type diffusion cell; IC_{50}: Half-maximal inhibitory concentration; MTS: CellTiter 96® AQ_{ueous} One Solution Cell Proliferation Assay (Promega); PBS: Phosphate-buffered saline; rpm: rounds per minute

Acknowledgments

The authors thank the Department of Pathology, University of Veterinary Medicine *Hannover* Foundation, Hannover, for providing equine thoracic skin for the FDC experiments. The authors thank the Institute for Anatomy, University of Veterinary Medicine Hannover, Foundation, Hannover, Germany for providing HE staining of equine thoracic skin.

Authors' contributions
LAW, JM, and JMVC designed the study, analyzed the data and drafted the manuscript. LAW performed cell culture and FDC experiments. JD performed statistical analysis of the data and aided in data analysis. JK developed and performed HPLC analysis. JuM developed the pharmaceutical test formulation. BP aided in cell culture experiments. KF, MK, AM, and RP aided in study design and data analysis. All authors read and approved the final manuscript.

Funding
The project was funded by the Central Innervation Programme from the German Federal Ministry for Economic Affairs and Energy.

Availability of data and materials
The datasets analyzed during the current study are available from the corresponding author on reasonable request.

Ethics approval and consent to participate
Not applicable.

Consent for publication
Not applicable.

Competing interests
Manfred Kietzmann is a member of the editorial board of BMC Veterinary Research.

Author details
[1]Clinic for Horses, University of Veterinary Medicine Hannover, Foundation, Bünteweg 9, 30559 Hannover, Germany. [2]Department of Pharmacology, Toxicology and Pharmacy, University of Veterinary Medicine Hannover, Foundation, Bünteweg 17, 30559 Hanover, Germany. [3]Biosolutions Halle GmbH, Weinbergweg 22, 06120 Halle (Saale), Germany. [4]Biozentrum, Martin Luther University Halle-Wittenberg, Weinbergweg 22, 06120 Halle (Saale), Germany. [5]Skinomics GmbH, Weinbergweg 23, 06120 Halle (Saale), Germany. [6]University Small Animal Clinic, University of Veterinary Medicine Vienna, Veterinärplatz 1, 1210 Vienna, Austria. [7]University Equine Clinic, University of Veterinary Medicine Vienna, Veterinärplatz 1, 1210 Vienna, Austria.

Received: 2 May 2019 Accepted: 24 January 2020
Published online: 05 February 2020

References
1. Kashiwada Y, Hashimoto F, Cosentino LM, Chen CH, Garrett PE, Lee KH. Betulinic acid and dihydrobetulinic acid derivatives as potent anti-HIV agents. J Med Chem. 1996;39:1016–7. https://doi.org/10.1021/jm950922q.
2. Enwerem NM, Okogun JI, Wambebe CO, Okorie DA, Akah PA. Anthelmintic activity of the stem bark extracts of Berlina grandiflora and one of its active principles, betulinic acid. Phytomedicine. 2001;8:112–4. https://doi.org/10.1078/0944-7113-00023.
3. Oliveira Costa JF, Barbosa-Filho JM, De Azevedo Maia GL, Guimarães ET, Meira CS, Ribeiro-Dos-Santos R, et al. Potent anti-inflammatory activity of betulinic acid treatment in a model of lethal endotoxemia. Int Immunopharmacol. 2014;23:469–74. https://doi.org/10.1016/j.intimp.2014.09.021.
4. Pisha E, Chai H, Lee I-S, Chagwedera TE, Farnsworth NHS, Cordell GA, et al. Discovery of betulinic acid as a selective inhibitor of human melanoma that functions by induction of apoptosis. Nat Med. 1995;1:1046–51. https://doi.org/10.1038/nm1095-1046.
5. Kessler JH, Mullauer FB, de Roo GM, Medema JP. Broad in vitro efficacy of plant-derived betulinic acid against cell lines derived from the most prevalent human cancer types. Cancer Lett. 2007;251:132–45. https://doi.org/10.1016/j.canlet.2006.11.003.
6. Rzeski W, Stepulak A, Szymański M, Sifringer M, Kaczor J, Wejksza K, et al. Betulinic acid decreases expression of bcl-2 and cyclin D1, inhibits proliferation, migration and induces apoptosis in cancer cells. Naunyn Schmiedeberg's Arch Pharmacol. 2006;374:11–20. https://doi.org/10.1007/s00210-006-0090-1.
7. Mullauer FB, Van Bloois L, Daalhuisen JB, Ten Brink MS, Storm G, Medema JP, et al. Betulinic acid delivered in liposomes reduces growth of human lung and colon cancers in mice without causing systemic toxicity. Anti-Cancer Drugs. 2011;22:223–33. https://doi.org/10.1097/CAD.0b013e3283421035.
8. Chintharlapalli S, Papineni S, Lei P, Pathi S, Safe S. Betulinic acid inhibits colon cancer cell and tumor growth and induces proteasome-dependent and -independent downregulation of specificity proteins (Sp) transcription factors. BMC Cancer. 2011;11:371. https://doi.org/10.1186/1471-2407-11-371.
9. Zhao J, Li R, Pawlak A, Henklewska M, Sysak A, Wen L, et al. Antitumor activity of betulinic acid and betulin in canine cancer cell lines. In Vivo (Brooklyn). 2018;32:1081–8. https://doi.org/10.21873/invivo.11349.
10. Wang W, Wang Y, Liu M, Zhang Y, Yang T, Li D, et al. Betulinic acid induces apoptosis and suppresses metastasis in hepatocellular carcinoma cell lines in vitro and in vivo. J Cell Mol Med. 2018:1–10. https://doi.org/10.1111/jcmm.13964.
11. Fulda S, Friesen C, Los M, Scaffidi C, Mier W, Benedict M, et al. Betulinic acid triggers CD95 (APO-1/Fas)- and p53-independent apoptosis via activation of caspases in neuroectodermal tumors. Cancer Res. 1997;57:4956–64.
12. Fulda S, Scaffidi G, Susin SA, Krammer PH, Kroemer G, Peter ME, et al. Activation of mitochondria and release of mitochondrial apoptogenic factors by betulinic acid. J Biol Chem. 1998;273:33942–8. https://doi.org/10.1074/jbc.273.51.33942.
13. Mullauer FB, Kessler JH, Medema JP. Betulinic acid induces cytochrome c release and apoptosis in a Bax/Bak-independent, permeability transition pore dependent fashion. Apoptosis. 2009;14:191–202. https://doi.org/10.1007/s10495-008-0290-x.
14. Raghuvar Gopal DV, Narkar AA, Badrinath Y, Mishra KP, Joshi DS. Protection of Ewing's sarcoma family tumor (ESFT) cell line SK-N-MC from betulinic acid induced apoptosis by α-DL-tocopherol. Toxicol Lett. 2004;153:201–12. https://doi.org/10.1016/j.toxlet.2004.03.027.
15. Tiwari R, Puthli A, Balakrishnan S, Sapra BK, Mishra KP. Betulinic acid-induced cytotoxicity in human breast tumor cell lines MCF-7 and T47D and its modification by tocopherol. Cancer Investig. 2014;32:402–8. https://doi.org/10.3109/07357907.2014.933234.
16. Tan YM, Yu R, Pezzuto JM. Betulinic acid-induced programmed cell death in human melanoma cells involves mitogen-activated protein kinase activation. Clin Cancer Res. 2003;9:2866–75.
17. Karna E, Szoka L, Palka JA. Betulinic acid inhibits the expression of hypoxia-inducible factor 1α and vascular endothelial growth factor in human endometrial adenocarcinoma cells. Mol Cell Biochem. 2010;340:15–20. https://doi.org/10.1007/s11010-010-0395-8.
18. Ren W, Qin L, Xu Y, Cheng N. Inhibition of betulinic acid to growth and angiogenesis of human colorectal cancer cell in nude mice. Chinese-German J Clin Oncol. 2010;9:153–7. https://doi.org/10.1007/s10330-010-0002-1.
19. Potze L, Mullauer FB, Colak S, Kessler JH, Medema JP. Betulinic acid-induced mitochondria-dependent cell death is counterbalanced by an autophagic salvage response. Cell Death Dis. 2014;5:e1169–8. https://doi.org/10.1038/cddis.2014.139.
20. Zuco V, Supino R, Righetti SC, Cleris L, Marchesi E, Gambacorti-Passerini C, et al. Selective cytotoxicity of betulinic acid on tumor cell lines, but not on normal cells. Cancer Lett. 2002;175:17–25. https://doi.org/10.1016/S0304-3835(01)00718-2.
21. Selzer E, Pimentel E, Wacheck V, Schlegel W, Pehamberger H, Jansen B, et al. Effects of betulinic acid alone and in combination with irradiation in human melanoma cells. J Invest Dermatol. 2000;114:935–40. https://doi.org/10.1046/j.1523-1747.2000.00972.x.
22. Potze L, Di Franco S, Grandela C, Pras-Raves ML, Picavet DI, Van Veen HA, et al. Betulinic acid induces a novel cell death pathway that depends on cardiolipin modification. Oncogene. 2016;35:427–37. https://doi.org/10.1038/onc.2015.102.
23. Liebscher G, Vanchangiri K, Mueller T, Feige K, Cavalleri JMV, Paschke R. In vitro anticancer activity of Betulinic acid and derivatives thereof on equine melanoma cell lines from grey horses and invivo safety assessment of the compound NVX-207 in two horses. Chem Biol Interact. 2016;246:20–9. https://doi.org/10.1016/j.cbi.2016.01.002.
24. McFadyean J. Equine melanomatosis. J Comp Pathol Ther. 1933;46:186–IN8. https://doi.org/10.1016/S0368-1742(33)80025-7.
25. Valentine BA. Equine melanocytic tumors: a retrospective study of 53 horses (1988 to 1991). J Vet Intern Med. 1995;9:291–7. https://doi.org/10.1111/j.1939-1676.1995.tb01087.x.

26. Moore JS, Shaw C, Shaw E, Buechner-Maxwell V, Scarratt WK, Crisman M, et al. Melanoma in horses: current perspectives. Equine Vet Educ. 2013;25: 144–51. https://doi.org/10.1111/j.2042-3292.2011.00368.x.
27. Rosengren Pielberg G, Golovko A, Sundström E, Curik I, Lennartsson J, Seltenhammer MH, et al. A cis-acting regulatory mutation causes premature hair graying and susceptibility to melanoma in the horse. Nat Genet. 2008; 40:1004–9. https://doi.org/10.1038/ng.185.
28. Sundström E, Komisarczuk AZ, Jiang L, Golovko A, Navratilova P, Rinkwitz S, et al. Identification of a melanocyte-specific, microphthalmia-associated transcription factor-dependent regulatory element in the intronic duplication causing hair greying and melanoma in horses. Pigment Cell Melanoma Res. 2012;25:28–36. https://doi.org/10.1111/j.1755-148X.2011.00902.x.
29. Seltenhammer MH, Simhofer H, Scherzer S, Zechner P, Curik I, Sölkner J, et al. Equine melanoma in a population of 296 grey Lipizzaner horses. Equine Vet J. 2010;35:153–7. https://doi.org/10.2746/042516403776114234.
30. Pilsworth RC, Knottenbelt DK. Melanoma. Equine Vet Educ. 2006;18:228–30. https://doi.org/10.2746/095777307X209194.
31. Macgillivray KC, Sweeney RW, Del PF. Metastatic Melanoma in Horses; 2002. p. 452–6.
32. Sundberg JP, Burnstein T, Page EH, Kirkham WWRF. Neoplasms of Equidae. J Am Vet Med Assoc. 1997;170:150–2 https://doi.org/10.137.
33. Scott D. Neoplastic diseases. In: Pedersen D, editor. Large Anim. Dermatology. Philadelphia: W.B. Saunders Company; 1988. p. 448–52.
34. Patterson-Kane JC, Sanchez LC, Uhl EW, Edens LM. Disseminated metastatic intramedullary melanoma in an aged grey horse. J Comp Pathol. 2001;125: 204–7. https://doi.org/10.1053/jcpa.2001.0481.
35. Borges IL, Lima TDS, Vale RG, Augusto P, Borges C, Batista S, et al. Metastatic cutaneous melanoma in equine: anatomopathological aspects. Artig Científico Med Veterinária Metastatic. 2017;11:32–8.
36. Metcalfe LV, O'Brien PJ, Papakonstantinou S, Cahalan SD, McAllister H, Duggan VE. Malignant melanoma in a grey horse: case presentation and review of equine melanoma treatment options. Ir Vet J. 2013;66:5. https://doi.org/10.1186/2046-0481-66-22.
37. Strauss RA, Allbaugh RA, Haynes J, Ben-Shlomo G. Primary corneal malignant melanoma in a horse. Equine Vet Educ. 2017:1–7. https://doi.org/10.1111/eve.12815.
38. Müller JMV, Feige K, Wunderlin P, Hödl A, Meli ML, Seltenhammer M, et al. Double-blind placebo-controlled study with interleukin-18 and interleukin-12-encoding plasmid DNA shows antitumor effect in metastatic melanoma in gray horses. J Immunother. 2011;34:58–64. https://doi.org/10.1097/CJI.0b013e3181fe1997.
39. Rowe EL, Sullins KE. Excision as treatment of dermal melanomatosis in horses: 11 cases (1994-2000). J Am Vet Med Assoc. 2004;225:94–6. https://doi.org/10.2460/javma.2004.225.94.
40. Groom LM, Sullins KE. Surgical excision of large melanocytic tumours in grey horses: 38 cases (2001–2013). Equine Vet Educ. 2018;30:438–43. https://doi.org/10.1111/eve.12767.
41. Théon AP, Wilson WD, Magdesian KG, Pusterla N, Snyder JR, Galuppo LD. Long-term outcome associated with intratumoral chemotherapy with cisplatin for cutaneous tumors in equidae: 573 cases (1995-2004). J Am Vet Med Assoc. 2007;230:1506–13. https://doi.org/10.2460/javma.230.10.1506.
42. Hewes CA, Sullins KE. Use of cisplatin-containing biodegradable beads for treatment of cutaneous neoplasia in equidae: 59 cases (2000-2004). J Am Vet Med Assoc. 2006;229:1617–22. https://doi.org/10.2460/javma.229.10.1617.
43. Mosmann T. Rapid colorimetric assay for cellular growth and survival: application to proliferation and cytotoxicity assays. J ImmunolMethods. 1983;65:55–63.
44. Scudiero D, McMahon J, Vistica D, Storeng R, Skehan P, Warren JT, et al. New colorimetric cytotoxicity assay for anticancer-drug screening. JNCI J Natl Cancer Inst. 2007;82:1107–12. https://doi.org/10.1093/jnci/82.13.1107.
45. Fulda S, Kroemer G. Targeting mitochondrial apoptosis by betulinic acid in human cancers. Drug Discov Today. 2009;14:885–90. https://doi.org/10.1016/j.drudis.2009.05.015.
46. Kommera H, Kaluderović GN, Kalbitz J, Paschke R. Lupane Triterpenoids-Betulin and Betulinic acid derivatives induce apoptosis in tumor cells. Investig New Drugs. 2011;29:266–72. https://doi.org/10.1007/s10637-009-9358-x.
47. Kommera H, Kaluderović GN, Dittrich S, Kalbitz J, Dräger B, Mueller T, et al. Carbamate derivatives of betulinic acid and betulin with selective cytotoxic activity. Bioorganic Med Chem Lett. 2010;20:3409–12. https://doi.org/10.1016/j.bmcl.2010.04.004.
48. Jiang L, Chen FX, Zang ST, Yang QF. Betulinic acid prevents high glucose-induced expression of extracellular matrix protein in cardiac fibroblasts by inhibiting the TGF-β1/Smad signaling pathway. Mol Med Rep. 2017;16: 6320–5. https://doi.org/10.3892/mmr.2017.7323.
49. Ali-Seyed M, Jantan I, Vijayaraghavan K, Bukhari SNA. Betulinic acid: recent advances in chemical modifications, effective delivery, and molecular mechanisms of a promising anticancer therapy. Chem Biol Drug Des. 2016; 87:517–36. https://doi.org/10.1111/cbdd.12682.
50. Smith SH, Goldschmidt MH, McManus PM. A comparative review of melanocytic neoplasms. Vet Pathol. 2002;39:651–78.
51. Seltenhammer MH, Heere-Ress E, Brandt S, Druml T, Jansen B, Pehamberger H, et al. Comparative histopathology of grey-horse-melanoma and human malignant melanoma. Pigment Cell Res. 2004;17:674–81. https://doi.org/10.1111/j.1600-0749.2004.00192.x.
52. Mills PC, Cross SE. Regional differences in transdermal penetration of hydrocortisone through equine skin. J Vet Pharmacol Ther. 2006;29:25–30. https://doi.org/10.1016/j.rvsc.2006.07.015.
53. Luís A, Ruela M, Perissinato AG, Esselin M, Lino DS. Evaluation of skin absorption of drugs from topical and transdermal formulations. Brazilian J Pharm Sci. 2016;52:527–44.
54. Dehelean CA, Feflea S, Ganta S, Amiji M. Anti-angiogenic effects of betulinic acid administered in nanoemulsion formulation using chorioallantoic membrane assay. J Biomed Nanotechnol. 2011;7:317–24. https://doi.org/10.1166/jbn.2011.1297.
55. Emmett MS, Dewing D, Pritchard-Jones RO. Angiogenesis and melanoma - from basic science to clinical trials. Am J Cancer Res. 2011;1:852–85268.
56. Huyke C, Reuter J, Rodig M, Kersten A, Laszczyk M, Scheffler A, et al. Treatment of actinic keratoses with a novel betulin-based oleogel. A prospective, randomized, comparative pilot study. J Der Dtsch Dermatologischen Gesellschaft. 2008;7:128–33. https://doi.org/10.1111/j.1610-0387.2008.06865.x.
57. Mählmann K. Minimalistic immunologically defined gene expression T helper cell 1 (MIDGE-Th1®) vectors coding for Interleukin 12 and −18 in combination with the transfection agent SAINT-18 have systemic antitumoral effects on equine melanomas, vol. 3: Cuvillier Verlag Göttingen; 2012.
58. Werner A, Braun M, Kietzmann M. Isolation and cultivation of canine corneal cells for in vitro studies on the anti-inflammatory effects of dexamethasone; 2008. p. 67–74.
59. Gillies RG, Didier N, Denton M. Determination of cell number in monolayer cultures. Anal Biochem. 1986;159:109–13.
60. Team RDC, R development Core Team R. R: A Language and Environment for Statistical Computing; 2008. https://doi.org/10.1007/978-3-540-74686-7.
61. Wood SN. Fast stable restricted maximum likelihood and marginal likelihood estimation of semiparametric generalized linear models. J R Stat Soc Ser B Stat Methodol. 2011;73:3–36. https://doi.org/10.1111/j.1467-9868.2010.00749.x.
62. Hothorn T, Bretz F, Westfall P. Simultaneous inference in general parametric models. Biom J. 2008;50:346–63. https://doi.org/10.1002/bimj.200810425.
63. Wickham H. Ggplot: elegant graphics for data analysis. J Stat Softw. 2010;35:1–3.

Publisher's Note

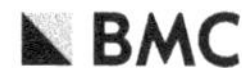

2.1. Supplemental data

Cell culture experiments

The cytotoxic (MTS assay) and antiproliferative (CVS assay) effects of BA were also tested on primary ES cells sRGO1 and sRGO2. ES cells were cultured under the same conditions as described for EMM cells eRGO1, but special cell culture flasks and 96-well plates were used (Nunc EasyFlask with Nunclon Delta Surface, ThermoFisher) and 15,000 cells/well were seeded for MTS assay. Information on the origin of the cells can be found in manuscript II. As even untreated sarcoid cells showed an altered growth behavior in 96 h experiments, proliferation and cytotoxicity experiments were performed only for 5, 24, and 48 h for this cell type.

cells	5 h	24 h	48 h
sRGO1	70.0 (58–82)	31.4 (21–41)	25.7 (11–41)
sRGO2	56.0 (43–70)	33.8 (6–61)	25.3 (15–36)

Table S1. IC_{50} values (µmol/L) of betulinic acid for primary equine sarcoid cells determined by MTS assay. Cytotoxic effects of betulinic acid on primary equine sarcoid cells (sRGO1 and sRGO2) after a treatment duration of 5, 24, or 48 h. Data represent mean IC_{50} values (µmol/L) of 6–8 independent experiments with 95% confidence interval in parentheses.

cells	5 h	24 h	48 h
sRGO1	44.6 (32–57)	25.5 (21–30)	21.7 (16–28)
sRGO2	n.a.	22.1 (18–26)	20,8 (17–24)

Table S2. IC_{50} values (µmol/L) of betulinic acid for primary equine sarcoid cells determined by CVS assay. Antiproliferative effects of betulinic acid on primary equine sarcoid cells (sRGO1 and sRGO2) after a treatment duration of 5, 24, or 48 h. Data represent mean IC_{50} values (µmol/L) of six independent experiments with 95% confidence interval in parentheses. n.a.= value not available (quantity of cells affected was too low to calculate an IC_{50} value with the software applied)

FDC experiments

Besides FDC experiments with an incubation time of 24 hours, permeation studies with an incubation time of 30 min were performed. The skin of six horses were used (two technical duplicates each). Because of the short incubation time in the 30-min-experiments, skin slices were pooled at 5 × 20 µm to investigate the concentration of BA/100 µm skin depth and, hence, increase the possibility to find amounts of BA above the HPLC detection limit (0.1 µg/mL). Otherwise, permeation studies, skin sample processing and HPLC analysis were performed as described in the manuscript.

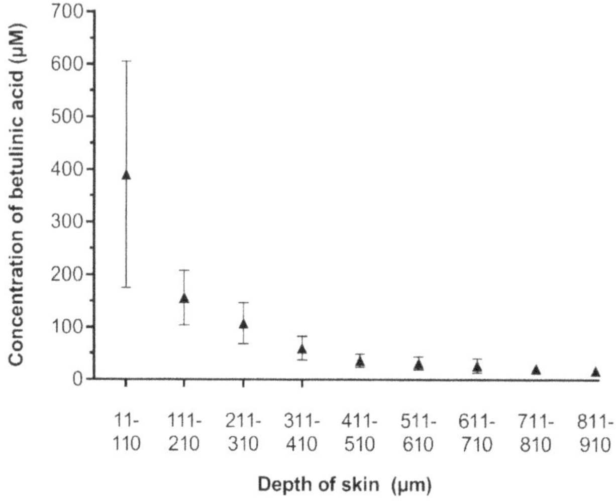

Figure S3. Concentration profile of BA correlative to skin thickness after 30 min of incubation. Figure data represent mean concentration (± SD) of BA in cryostat skin slices at different skin depths determined by high-performance liquid chromatography.

3. Manuscript II:

In vitro assessment of triterpenoids NVX-207 and betulinyl-bis-sulfamate as a topical treatment for equine skin cancer

Lisa A. Weber[1], Anne Funtan[2], Reinhard Paschke[2], Julien Delarocque[1], Jutta Kalbitz[3], Jessica Meißner[4], Karsten Feige[1], Manfred Kietzmann[4], Jessika-M.V. Cavalleri[5*]

[1] Clinic for Horses, University of Veterinary Medicine Hannover, Foundation, Bünteweg 9, 30559 Hannover, Germany

[2] Biozentrum, Martin-Luther-University Halle-Wittenberg, Weinbergweg 22, 06120 Halle (Saale), Germany

[3] Biosolutions Halle GmbH, Weinbergweg 22, 06120 Halle (Saale), Germany

[4] Department of Pharmacology, Toxicology and Pharmacy, University of Veterinary Medicine Hannover, Foundation, Bünteweg 17, 30559 Hannover, Germany

[5] Equine Internal Medicine, University Equine Clinic, University of Veterinary Medicine Vienna, Veterinärplatz 1, 1210 Vienna, Austria

[*] Corresponding author

PLOS ONE 2020;15(11):1-22

Accepted: 14 October 2020, published online: 05 November 2020

DOI: 10.1371/journal.pone.0241448

Contribution to the manuscript:

LAW: study design, investigation (CVS and MTS assay, FDC experiments, skin sample processing for HPLC analysis), data analysis, project administration, visualization, manuscript drafting and editing; AF: study design, investigation (apoptosis tests), data analysis, visualization, manuscript editing; RP: study design, funding requisition, project administration, supervision of AF; JD: formal analysis, visualization; JK: investigation (HPLC analysis), methodology; JM: study design, funding requisition, resources, supervision of LAW; KF: funding requisition, supervision of LAW; MK: data analysis, resources, supervision of LAW; JMVC: study design, funding requisition, project administration, manuscript review, supervision of LAW. All authors read and approved the final manuscript.

PLOS ONE

RESEARCH ARTICLE

In vitro assessment of triterpenoids NVX-207 and betulinyl-bis-sulfamate as a topical treatment for equine skin cancer

Lisa Annabel Weber[1], Anne Funtan[2], Reinhard Paschke[2], Julien Delarocque[1], Jutta Kalbitz[3], Jessica Meißner[4], Karsten Feige[1], Manfred Kietzmann[4], Jessika-Maximiliane V. Cavalleri[5]*

1 Clinic for Horses, University of Veterinary Medicine Hannover, Foundation, Hannover, Germany, **2** Biozentrum, Martin-Luther-University Halle-Wittenberg, Halle (Saale), Germany, **3** BioSolutions Halle GmbH, Halle (Saale), Germany, **4** Department of Pharmacology, Toxicology and Pharmacy, University of Veterinary Medicine Hannover, Foundation, Hannover, Germany, **5** Equine Internal Medicine, University Equine Clinic, University of Veterinary Medicine Vienna, Vienna, Austria

* Jessika.Cavalleri@vetmeduni.ac.at

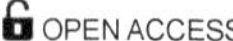

Citation: Weber LA, Funtan A, Paschke R, Delarocque J, Kalbitz J, Meißner J, et al. (2020) *In vitro* assessment of triterpenoids NVX-207 and betulinyl-bis-sulfamate as a topical treatment for equine skin cancer. PLoS ONE 15(11): e0241448. https://doi.org/10.1371/journal.pone.0241448

Editor: Irina V. Lebedeva, Columbia University, UNITED STATES

Received: May 1, 2020

Accepted: October 14, 2020

Published: November 5, 2020

Peer Review History: PLOS recognizes the benefits of transparency in the peer review process; therefore, we enable the publication of all of the content of peer review and author responses alongside final, published articles. The editorial history of this article is available here: https://doi.org/10.1371/journal.pone.0241448

Data Availability Statement: All relevant data are within the manuscript and its Supporting information files.

Abstract

Equine sarcoid (ES) is the most prevalent skin tumor in equids worldwide. Additionally, aging grey horses frequently suffer from equine malignant melanoma (EMM). Current local therapies targeting these skin tumors remain challenging. Therefore, more feasible topical treatment options should be considered. In order to develop a topical therapy against ES and EMM, betulinyl-bis-sulfamate and NVX-207, derivatives of the naturally occurring betulin and betulinic acid, respectively, were evaluated for their antiproliferative (crystal violet staining assay), cytotoxic (MTS assay) and apoptotic (AnnexinV staining, cell cycle investigations) effects on primary ES cells, EMM cells and equine dermal fibroblasts *in vitro.* The more potent derivative was assessed for its *in vitro* penetration and permeation on isolated equine skin within 30 min and 24 h using Franz-type diffusion cells and HPLC analysis. Betulinyl-bis-sulfamate and NVX-207 inhibited the proliferation and metabolism in ES cells, EMM cells and fibroblasts significantly ($p < 0.001$) in a time- and dose-dependent manner. NVX-207 had superior anticancer effects compared to betulinyl-bis-sulfamate. Both compounds led to the externalization of phosphatidylserines on the cell membrane and DNA fragmentation, demonstrating that the effective mode of action was apoptosis. After 48 h of treatment with NVX-207, the number of necrotic cells was less than 2% in all cell types. Detected amounts of NVX-207 in the different skin layers exceeded the half-maximal inhibitory concentrations calculated by far. Even though data obtained *in vitro* are auspicious, the results are not unconditionally applicable to the clinical situation. Consequently, *in vivo* studies are required to address the antitumoral effects of topically applied NVX-207 in ES and EMM patients.

Funding: Some authors were funded by the Central Innovation Programme of the German Federal Ministry for Economic Affairs and Energy. LAW: Specific grant number: TopiDrugHorse 16KN051526 BMWI; AF: Specific grant number: TopiDrugHorse 16KN051530 BMWI; RP: Specific grant number: TopiDrugHorse 16KN051524 BMWI; JK: Specific grant number: TopiDrugHorse 16KN051524 BMWI. RP and JK were further funded by BioSolutions Halle GmbH (www.biosolutions-halle.de). The TopiDrugHorse project is a cooperation project between research institutions and a company. The participation of a company in this cooperation project is the prerequisite for the approval of the project funds by the Ministry of Economic Affairs and Energy. BioSolutions Halle GmbH is therefore not a commercial funder, but an equal partner. The rights and obligations of all partners are governed by a cooperation agreement. This applies in particular to publications and intellectual property. The funders provided support in the form of salaries and/or research materials for authors [LAW, AF, RP, JK], but did not have any additional role in the study design, data collection and analysis, decision to publish, or preparation of the manuscript. The specific roles of these authors are articulated in the 'author contributions' section.

Competing interests: The authors declare that no competing interests exist. The affiliation "BioSolutions Halle GmbH" of Dr. Jutta Kalbitz does not alter our adherence to PLOS ONE policies on sharing data and materials. As described in the Funding Statement, BioSolutions Halle GmbH is not a commercial funder, but an equal partner in the TopiDrugHorse project.

Introduction

The skin is the organ in horses most frequently affected by tumors [1]. With a reported occurrence ranging from 35 to 90% of all cutaneous neoplasms [2–4], the equine sarcoid (ES) is the most prevalent skin cancer in equids worldwide [5–7]. The pathogenesis of this coat-color independent tumor of the fibroblasts has been linked to an infection with the bovine papillomavirus type 1 and 2 [8–10], trauma [11, 12], and a genetic predisposition [13, 14]. According to their gross appearance and clinical behavior, sarcoids are classified into six types: Mild occult or verrucous tumors and more severe nodular, fibroblastic, mixed and malevolent lesions [12]. Even though non-metastasizing and mostly not life-threatening, their locally invasive growth and predilection sites (e.g. head, saddle girth area) can seriously impair the equid's welfare and compromise the use and economic value of the animal [1]. Multiple treatment modalities for the ES are described in the literature (e.g. surgery, radiation, chemotherapy, immunotherapy) but universal effectiveness is not given and recurrence rates are high [11, 15]. Topical therapies generally seem particularly feasible as they are noninvasive and applicable, even on treatment sites that are difficult to access. However, the results regarding the efficacy of the acyclovir cream often used for mild-type ES treatment are contradictory [16, 17] and imiquimod may temporarily cause severe local side effects [18]. In addition, although a variety of other topical treatment options exists, mainly anecdotal evidence of their success is reported [1, 15, 19, 20]. Therefore, the development of a novel topical treatment approach for ES should be considered to take advantage of the benefits of topical therapies.

The equine malignant melanoma (EMM) is a frequently occurring, sex-independent skin neoplasm with a high prevalence in grey horses older than 15 years of age [21–25]. Melanomas are melanocytic tumors which typically occur as nodular in glabrous cutaneous regions (e.g. ventral surface of the tail, perineum, anus, external genitalia) [22, 26]. The dominant age-related phenotype of greying and the predisposition to melanoma are associated with a mutation in intron 6 of the syntaxin-17 gene [27, 28]. Most of the tumors show a slow growth pattern over years, however, more than 60% become malignant and cause clinical problems due to enlargement und widespread metastases [29–31]. Treatment options reported with varying outcomes include systemic and local approaches, such as immunotherapy [32–34], cimetidine application [35, 36], radiation [37], surgery [38, 39], and chemotherapy with cisplatin alone [40, 41] or in combination with electrochemotherapy [42, 43]. Although effective in many cases, surgical excision can be challenging due to the unfavorable localization of the tumors and the intratumoral injection of the mutagenic and carcinogenic cisplatin is linked to strict safety rules [44]. Therefore, a more practical treatment option for early stages of EMM, for example, in the form of a cream, would be useful.

Promising substances for topical ES and EMM treatment could be triterpenoids, such as betulinic acid (BA) and its derivatives [45, 46]. Betulinic acid, the oxidation product of betulin, is a pentacyclic lupane-type triterpenoid and can be extracted from various botanical sources [47]. Since first studies proved BA's antitumor activity against human melanoma and other malignancies in cell culture and animal models [48, 49], a plethora of scientific work has verified the wide range of its biological capabilities *in vitro* and *in vivo* [50, 51]. Treatment with BA induces apoptosis in cancer cells due to a direct effect on the mitochondria [52] independent of CD95 ligand/receptor interaction [49]. Alterations in the mitochondrial membrane potential mediate a cytochrome *c* and apoptosis-inducing factor release, which results in the cleavage of caspases and nuclear disintegration [53, 54]. Furthermore, the generation of reactive oxygen species [49, 55], the subsequent mitogen-activated protein kinase activation [56] and the inhibition of eukaryotic topoisomerase I [57], endothelial-to-mesenchymal-transition [58] and angiogenesis [59, 60] are suggested as BA-mediated antitumoral properties. The anticancer effects of BA against EMM cells and its potent permeation in isolated equine skin have recently been reported [45]. However, based on a classification for the cytotoxicity of triterpenes [61], the half-maximal inhibitory concentrations (IC_{50}) of BA for EMM cells and other human and animal cancer cell lines are considered to be only moderate. In addition, the compounds' hydrosolubility is limited, which reduces the opportunities of medicinal use mainly to topical applications [62]. A variety of synthetically modified derivatives have been synthesized in the past few decades to enhance the pharmacological properties of BA and the closely related compound betulin [62]. Among these are betulinyl-bis-sulfamate ((3β)-Lup-20(29)-ene-3,28-diol, 3,28-disulfamate; BBS) [63] and NVX-207 (3-acetyl-betulinic acid-2-amino-3-hydroxy-2-hydroxymethyl-propanoate) [64], from which, especially the latter substance, shows a higher cytotoxicity in various human and canine cancer cell lines compared to the parent BA [64–66]. It has been demonstrated that NVX-207 induces apoptosis in EMM cells [66]. In addition, the compound has already been successfully tested in a clinical study with canine cancer patients [64]. Within the frame of pilot safety studies, NVX-207 was well tolerated when applied topically in eight healthy horses [67] or injected intralesionally in two horses affected by EMM [66].

The objectives of this study were (1) to investigate the betulin derivative BBS and BA derivative NVX-207 for their antiproliferative, cytotoxic and apoptotic effects on ES cells, EMM cells and equine dermal fibroblasts and (2) to assess the more potent derivative for its penetration and permeation on isolated equine skin *in vitro* with the aim of developing a topical therapy for the ES and EMM.

Material and methods

Evaluation of the anticancer effects of BBS and NVX-207 on equine melanoma cells and equine dermal fibroblasts

Compounds. Biosolutions Halle GmbH (Halle/Saale, Germany) synthesized BBS and NVX-207. The compounds were dissolved in dimethyl sulfoxide (WAK-Chemie Medical GmbH, Steinbach, Germany) to achieve 20 mM stock solutions.

Cells and culture conditions. All cells used for the experiments originate from different horses. Primary EMM cells (MelDuWi) and primary equine dermal fibroblasts (PriFi1, PriFi2) belong to the cell culture stock of the Clinic for Horses, University of Veterinary Medicine Hannover, Foundation, Hannover, Germany. The cells were cultured as monolayers at 37°C in a humified atmosphere with 5% CO_2 and maintained in RPMI1640 cell culture medium with stable glutamine (Biochrom GmbH, Berlin, Germany) supplemented with 15% fetal bovine serum superior (Biochrom GmbH) and 1% penicillin and streptomycin (10,000 international units (I.U.)/mL /10,000 μg/mL, Biochrom GmbH). Primary ES cells sRGO1 and sRGO2 (kindly provided by Dr. Sabine Brandt, University of Veterinary Medicine Vienna, Vienna, Austria) and primary EMM cells eRGO1 (kindly provided by Dr. Barbara Pratscher, University of Veterinary Medicine Vienna, Vienna, Austria) were cultured as monolayers at 37°C in a humified atmosphere with 5% CO_2 and kept in Dulbecco's modified Eagle's high glucose w/Glutamax (4.5 g/L) cell culture medium (GIBCO-Invitrogen, Thermofisher, Darmstadt, Germany) supplemented with 10% fetal bovine serum superior (Biochrom GmbH) and 1% Antibiotic-Antimycotic (100x; GIBCO-Invitrogen), containing penicillin (10,000 units/mL), streptomycin (10,000 μg/mL) and amphotericin B (25 μg/mL).

Proliferation assay. The proliferation assay was performed as published [45]. Briefly, a modified crystal violet staining assay (CVS) was carried out to investigate the antiproliferative effects of BBS and NVX-207 on primary equine cells. The cells were exposed to BBS and NVX-207 at nine different concentrations ranging from 1–100 μmol/L for 5, 24, 48 and 96 h.

Proliferation and cytotoxicity experiments for this cell type were performed only for 5, 24 and 48 h as even untreated sarcoid cells showed an altered growth behavior in 96 h experiments. Control cells were treated with medium only. The proportion of cells treated relative to untreated controls was determined by crystal violet staining and photometric absorbance measurement at the incubation time points mentioned above. Proliferation assays were performed in six to eight biological replicates with two technical replicates for each combination of cell type, incubation time and compound concentration.

Cytotoxicity assay. The cytotoxicity of the compounds was assessed by the CellTiter 96® AQ_{ueous} One Solution Cell Proliferation Assay (MTS) (Promega GmbH, Mannheim, Germany) as reported [45]. In brief, in order to reach cell confluence within 48 h, cells were seeded into 96-well plates in adequate densities (MelDuWi 30,000 cells/well; PriFi1, PriFi2, eRGO1 20,000 cells/well; sRGO1and sRGO2 15,000 cells/well). Incubation times and concentrations of BBS and NVX-207 were applied in accordance with the CVS assay. The formazan dye generated by the metabolic active cells was quantified photometrically. Cytotoxicity assays were performed in six to nine biological replicates with two technical replicates for each combination of cell type, incubation time and compound concentration.

Cell cycle investigations. Approximately 7.5×10^5 cells (MelDuWi) and 1.0×10^6 cells (PriFri2 and sRGO2) were seeded in 25 cm^2 cell culture flasks. After 24 h of incubation, the medium was replaced with medium containing either BBS or NVX-207 at their respective double IC_{50} concentration (measured after 96 h by sulforhodamine B [SRB] assay, analogous to [66]; see S1 and S2 Appendices). Following 24 and 48 h of incubation, the cells were harvested by mild trypsinization and washed twice with phosphate-buffered saline (PBS) buffer (containing Mg^{2+} and Ca^{2+}). Cells (1.0×10^6) were fixed with ethanol (70%, -20°C, for 24 h). After discarding the ethanol, the cells were washed in 1 mL PBS buffer (containing Mg^{2+} and Ca^{2+}) and were centrifuged. The cell pellet was resuspended in 1 mL of staining PBS buffer (containing Mg^{2+} and Ca^{2+}, 10 μg/mL RNASe [Thermofisher] and 15 μg/mL propidium iodide [Sigma-Aldrich, Munich, Germany]) and was incubated for 30 min at room temperature. Analyses were performed using the Attune® FACS machine (Life Technologies, Darmstadt, Germany) collecting data from the BL-2A channel. Doublet cells were excluded from the measurements by plotting BL-2A against BL-2H. A total of 20,000 events were collected for each cell cycle distribution. Each sample was measured in duplicate.

AnnexinV staining. Approximately 7.5×10^5 cells (MelDuWi) and 1.0×10^6 cells (PriFri2 and sRGO2) were seeded in 25 cm^2 cell culture flasks. After 24 h of incubation, the medium was replaced with medium containing either BBS or NVX-207 at their respective double IC_{50} concentration (measured after 96 h). Following 24 and 48 h of incubation, cells were harvested by mild trypsinization and washed twice with PBS buffer (containing Mg^{2+} and Ca^{2+}). Cells (1.0×10^6) were resuspended in AnnexinV binding buffer (BioLegend®, San Diego, US) to a concentration of $1.0 \cdot 10^6$ cells/mL. Approximately 100,000 cells were stained with propidium iodide solution (3 mL, 1 mg/mL) and FITC AnnexinV solution (5 mL, BioLegend®) for 15 min in the dark at room temperature. After the addition of Annexin V binding buffer (400 mL), the suspension was analyzed using the Attune® FACS machine (Life Technologies). After gating for living cells, the data from detectors BL-1A and BL-3A were collected. A total of 20,000 events were collected from each sample and technical duplicates were measured.

Diffusion of NVX-207 into equine skin

Test formulations. Two different pharmaceutical formulations were provided by Skinomics GmbH, Halle, Germany, for *in vitro* permeation studies. Based on previous permeation studies with BA [45], test formulation 1 consisted of "Basiscreme DAC" (pharmaceutical

Table 1. Information about the equine skin donors used for Franz-type diffusion cell experiments.

Incubation time	Number of horses	Sex	Breed	Median age in years (range min-max)
30 min	6	3 mares, 2 geldings, 1 unknown	1 Hanoverian Warmblood, 1 Icelandic horse, 1 Arabian horse, 1 Clydesdale, 2 unknown	19 (4–23)
24 h	6	2 mares, 4 geldings	2 Warmblood horses, 1 Hanoverian Warmblood, 1 Holsteiner Warmblood, 1 Arabian horse, 1 Icelandic horse	16 (6–25)

https://doi.org/10.1371/journal.pone.0241448.t001

amphiphilic cream as published in the German Drug Codex) with 1% NVX-207 and 20% medium-chain triglycerides. The formulation was modified because of an inhomogenous distribution of NVX-207 in test formulation 1 (oily sediments and overall recovery rate < 50% in Franz-type diffusion cells (FDC) experiments): Test formulation 2 contained "Basiscreme DAC" with 1% NVX-207.

Skin sample preparation and Franz-type diffusion cell experiments. Skin from six horses was used for each FDC experiment. The skin from the lateral thorax was dissected at the Institute of Pathology, University of Veterinary Medicine Hannover, Foundation, Hannover, Germany, after euthanasia of the horses at the Clinic for Horses, University of Veterinary Medicine Hannover, Foundation, for reasons unrelated to the present study. Therefore, a prospective approval of the experiments by an animal research ethics committee was not required. Skin samples were stored at -20°C until use (maximum five months). Table 1 provides information about the sex, breed and age of the different equine skin donors. Further skin sample preparation and diffusion experiments were performed as reported [45]. Skin samples were incubated with test formulation 1 for 24 h and with test formulation 2 for 30 min and 24 h, respectively.

Sample processing and NVX-207 quantification. Following diffusion experiments, skin sample processing and NVX-207 quantification were performed as published with a few modifications [45]. In short, in order to determine the concentration of NVX-207 in different skin layers, skin samples were cut with a cryostat (CryoStar™ NX70 Cryostat, Thermofisher, Darmstadt, Germany) in slices parallel to the skin surface starting from the epidermal side. The first slice had a thickness of 10 μm and, therefore, included the *stratum corneum* with potential residues of the test formulation, which had not been removed with the cotton swab. The following slices were 20-μm thick. Because of the short incubation time in the experiments (30 min), slices were pooled at 5 × 20 μm to investigate the concentration of NVX-207/100 μm skin depth and, therefore, increase the possibility of finding amounts of NVX-207 above the detection limit (0.1 μg/mL). A higher permeation rate of the compound was expected for 24-h experiments and, therefore, the 20-μm slices were stored and analyzed separately up to a depth of 310 μm. The slices were then pooled at 5 × 20 μm until a depth of a maximal 910 μm was reached. The cryostat blade was cleaned with tissues soaked in 80% methanol between each cut. The quantity of NVX-207 was determined by an analytic high-performance liquid chromatography (HPLC) method. Reverse phase analysis was performed using an Agilent 1100 system (Agilent, Waldbronn, Germany) on a Luna® Omega column (3 μm, PS C18, 100 Å, 150 x 4.6 mm; Phenomenex, Torrance, US) at 30°C using a gradient method with acetonitrile (0.1% HCOOH)(A):water (0.1% HCOOH)(B) at 1.1 mL/min, (from 60 to 10% B within 7.50 min). The diode array detector was set at 200 nm.

Statistical analysis

Technical duplicates with a coefficient of variation of more than 20% were excluded from the cell assay analysis. IC_{50} values of BBS and NVX-207 from the proliferation and cytotoxicity tests were calculated with the pharmacodynamic model 108 of Phoenix® WinNonlin® software (version 8.1, Certara, USA). Additional statistical data analysis was conducted with R 3.5.1. [68]. A generalized additive model was fitted for each test (MTS and CVS) and cell type comparison (primary EMM cells and fibroblasts, and primary ES cells and fibroblasts) using the 'mgcv' package [69]. Compound concentrations and the duration of incubation were modeled as tensor product smooth interacting with compound and cell line. Cell passage was added as a random effect. An appropriate distribution was selected by the visual inspection of residuals. The p-values were obtained by performing a Wald test for each parameter. Statistical significance was set at 0.05.

Results

Proliferation inhibition and cytotoxicity of BBS and NVX-207 on equine cells

The antiproliferative and cytotoxic effects of NVX-207 and BBS on ES cells, EMM cells and equine dermal fibroblasts were assessed by the CVS and MTS assay. In general, both compounds had significant inhibitory effects on cell proliferation ($p < 0.001$ in CVS assay for every cell type) and cell viability ($p < 0.001$ in MTS assay for every cell type) compared to untreated controls. However, effects on the cells were dose- and time-dependent. Figs 1 and 2 show the results from the melanoma cell model. Results of the sarcoid cell model are attached as additional files S3 and S4 Appendices. First significant, dose-dependent antiproliferative effects on ES cells, EMM cells and fibroblasts were observed after 24 h of incubation with BBS and after 5 h of incubation with NVX-207. A significant, dose-dependent reduction in cell viability was observed in ES cells, EMM cells and fibroblasts after 5 h of treatment with BBS and NVX-207.

As assessed by determination of IC_{50} values (Table 2) NVX-207 was more active against the investigated equine cells compared to BBS. When the cells were exposed to BBS for 5 h, the quantity of cells affected was too low to calculate the IC_{50} values in both cytotoxicity and proliferation assays. After 48 h, NVX-207 exceeded BBSs' antiproliferative effects about 23 and 29 times in ES cells sRGO1 and sRGO2, respectively, about 25 and 3 times in EMM cells eRGO1 and MelDuWi, respectively, and about 23 and 6 times in fibroblasts PriFi1 and PriFi2, respectively. NVX-207 was about 11 (sRGO1), 25 (sRGO2), 8 (eRGO1), 3 (MelDuWi), 34 (PriFi1) and 9 (PriFi2) times more cytotoxic than BBS.

Selectivity of both compounds towards the different cells varied. Compared to normal fibroblasts, BBS showed a selectivity to both sarcoid and EMM cells in the proliferation assay and a selectivity to eRGO1 and both sarcoid cell types in the cytotoxicity assay. Sarcoid cells were more sensitive to BBS than EMM cells. Normal fibroblasts did not show a better tolerance towards NVX-207 compared to EMM cells; by contrast, MelDuWi were revealed to be more resistant in both assays. A selectivity of NVX-207 towards fibroblasts was observed in the proliferation assay for sarcoid cells.

Cell cycle investigations. The cell death mechanisms of NVX-207 and BBS on ES cells, EMM cells and equine dermal fibroblasts were assessed by cell cycle investigations via flow cytometry. Condensation of chromatin and fragmentation of DNA and nuclei occurs in apoptotic cells, which can be detected by the SubG1 peak. In comparison to untreated cells (control), the treatment with BBS and NVX-207 caused an increase of subG1 cells after 48 h of treatment for all equine cells (Fig 3 and S5–S12 Appendices). The subG1 peak for the EMM cells MelDuWi arose after a treatment of 48 h to more than 40% for BBS and more than 60% for NVX-207. The equine dermal fibroblasts PriFi2 also showed an increased numbers of subG1 cells (> 80%) after 48 h of treatment with NVX-207 but only 14% after 48 h of

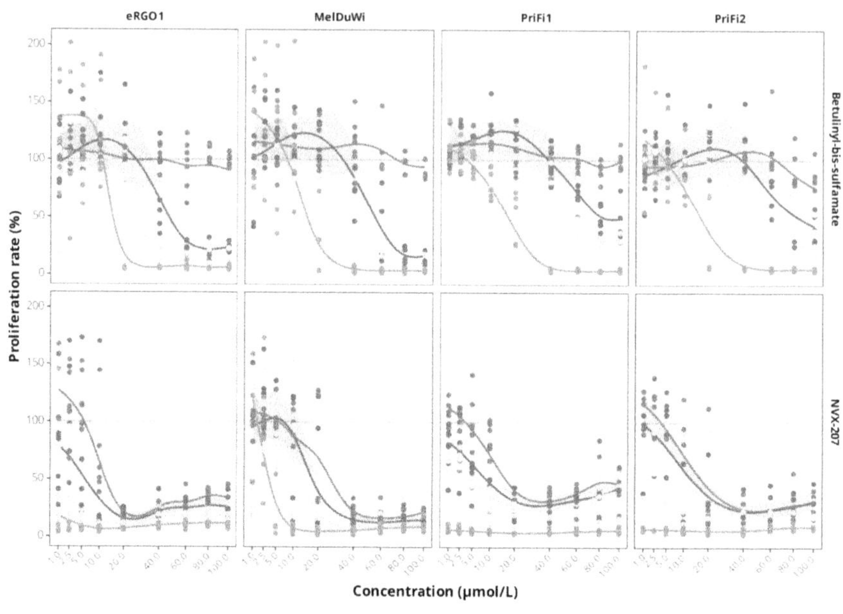

Fig 1. Effects of betulinyl-bis-sulfamate and NVX-207 on primary equine cell proliferation at different time points. Proliferation dose-response regression lines of betulinyl-bis-sulfamate (BBS) and NVX-207 on primary equine malignant melanoma (EMM) cells (eRGO1, MelDuWi) and primary equine dermal fibroblasts (PriFi1, PriFi2) at four different time points (5, 24, 48 and 96 h) determined by CVS assay. Antiproliferative effects of the compounds on primary equine cells increase with the concentration and time of drug exposition. Data represent regression lines and 95% confidence intervals of 6–8 independent experiments for each combination of cell type, incubation time and concentration. Concentrations at which the corresponding 95% confidence intervals do not cross the 100% line indicate a significant reduction of the proliferation rate.

https://doi.org/10.1371/journal.pone.0241448.g001

treatment with BBS (Fig 4 and S12 Appendix). Thus, a selectivity of BBS for the initiation of the preferably programmed cell death in EMM cells could be shown. The effect of both active substances on the sarcoid cells was noticeably lower compared to the other cell lines. After a treatment time of 48 h, an enrichment of 20% subG1 cells was present.

AnnexinV staining. The externalization of phosphatidylserines to the extracellular side of the plasma membrane is a characteristic and early event in apoptosis [70, 71]. The change of the extracellular plasma membrane composition was detected by using AnnexinV-FITC/ (propidium iodide) staining and analysis by flow cytometry (Figs 5 and 6 and S13–S20 Appendices). Untreated cells were used for control. After a treatment period of 24 h with BBS, 19% of the sarcoid cells were early apoptotic and 39% were late apoptotic, while 2% of the control cells were early and 14% were late apoptotic. After 48 h, the number of apoptotic cells further increased and approximately 90% of the cells were apoptotic (8% early apoptotic; 82% late apoptotic). NVX-207 had a weaker effect on the sarcoid cells and 40% were present as living cells after 48 h. The equine dermal fibroblasts showed a slower increase of apoptotic cells after 24 h of treatment with BBS. In this case, increases of 5% early apoptotic and 3% late apoptotic cells

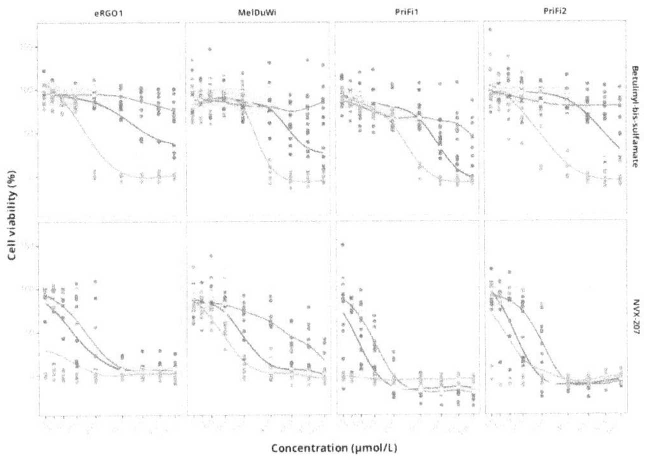

Fig 2. Effects of betulinyl-bis-sulfamate and NVX-207 on primary equine cell viability at different time points. Cytotoxicity dose-response regression lines of BBS and NVX-207 on primary EMM cells (eRGO1, MelDuWi) and primary equine dermal fibroblasts (PriFi1, PriFi2) at four different time points (5, 24, 48 and 96 h) determined by MTS assay. Cytotoxic effects of the compounds on primary equine cells increase with concentration and time of drug exposition. Data represent regression lines and 95% confidence intervals of 6–9 independent experiments for each combination of cell type, incubation time and concentration. Concentrations at which the corresponding 95% confidence intervals do not cross the 100% line indicate a significant reduction of cell viability.

https://doi.org/10.1371/journal.pone.0241448.g002

were present. However, an increase in late apoptotic cells after 48 h was observed (54% by treatment with BBS and 67% with NVX-207). Thus, it was shown that BBS had a better selectivity to sarcoid cells compared to fibroblasts.

Compared to BBS, NVX-207 had the stronger potential to induce apoptosis in EMM cells. After 48 h, 45% were late apoptotic cells and only 30% were living cells. In addition, 25% of cells were present in the early apoptotic phase. It was proven for all three equine cell lines that the necrosis rate after 48 h of treatment with NVX-207 was below 2%.

Diffusion of NVX-207 into equine skin and overall NVX-207 recoveries

When the skin samples were treated with test formulation 2 for 30 min, NVX-207 was detected in both the epidermis and dermis (Fig 7). An incubation time of 24 h led to an accumulation of the compound in the upper epidermis (11–30 μm) but did not increase the amount of NVX-207 in the other skin layers analyzed (Fig 7 and S21 Appendix). The detected concentrations exceeded the 24 h IC_{50} values of NVX-207 for ES cells, EMM cells and equine dermal fibroblasts determined in the proliferation and cytotoxicity assays even in the deeper skin layers examined (up to a depth of 810 μm). The overall NVX-207 recovery rate after 30 min of incubation was 89 ± 23% (mean ± SD; n = 6), from which 68 ± 18% of the substance was detected in the non-permeated proportion (cotton swabs) and 28 ± 17% in the skin. The overall recovery rate of NVX-207 in test formulation 2 after 24 h of incubation was 85 ± 14% (mean ± SD; n = 6). A quantity of 51 ± 9% of the NVX-207 amount applied was found in the

Table 2. IC_{50} values (µmol/L) of betulinyl-bis-sulfamate (BBS) and NVX-207 for primary equine cells determined by CVS and MTS assay after 5, 24, 48 and 96 h of drug exposure.

		5 h		
		Compound and assay		
	BBS		**NVX-207**	
Cells	**CVS**	**MTS**	**CVS**	**MTS**
sRGO1	-	-	7 (5–10)	9 (7–11)
sRGO2	-	-	6 (4–8)	8 (6–11)
eRGO1	-	-	10 (7–13)	9 (4–15)
MelDuWi	-	-	20 (13–26)	-
PriFi1	-	-	11 (-2–23)	11 (9–13)
PriFi2	-	-	14 (4–24)	20 (18–22)
		24 h		
		Compound and assay		
	BBS		**NVX-207**	
Cells	**CVS**	**MTS**	**CVS**	**MTS**
sRGO1	40 (31–49)	-	7 (5–10)	4 (2–5)
sRGO2	38 (33–43)	45 (40–49)	< 1 (0–2)	3 (2–4)
eRGO1	42 (36–48)	47 (37–57)	5 (3–7)	7 (4–15)
MelDuWi	50 (38–61)	60 (30–91)	16 (11–21)	18 (15–21)
PriFi1	52 (41–62)	59 (50–68)	4 (2–6)	4 (2–5)
PriFi2	62 (48–76)	77 (35–118)	8 (4–12)	7 (5–9)
		48 h		
		Compound and assay		
	BBS		**NVX-207**	
Cells	**CVS**	**MTS**	**CVS**	**MTS**
sRGO1	23 (16–31)	25 (21–30)	< 1 (0–1)	2 (1–4)
sRGO2	29 (19–31)	28 (21–35)	< 1 (< 0–8)	1 (< 1–2)
eRGO1	25 (7–44)	32 (26–38)	< 1 (< 0 –< 1)	4 (1–7)
MelDuWi	36 (26–46)	53 (41–65)	12 (6–18)	15 (12–19)
PriFi1	42 (32–51)	35 (31–39)	2 (1–3)	1 (< 1–2)
PriFi2	39 (32–46)	61 (48–74)	7 (< 0–15)	7 (< 1–7)
		96 h		
		Compound and assay		
	BBS		**NVX-207**	
Cells	**CVS**	**MTS**	**CVS**	**MTS**
sRGO1	n.a.	n.a.	n.a.	n.a.
sRGO2	n.a.	n.a.	n.a.	n.a.
eRGO1	15 (5–25) 0.04)	16 (13–18)	< 1 (< 0 –	< 1 (< 0 –< 1)
MelDuWi	16 (4–29)	32 (15–49)	4 (3–5)	8 (5–10)
PriFi1	17 (15–20)	28 (26–31)	< 1 (< 0 –< 1)	< 1 (< 0 –< 1)
PriFi2	16 (11–21)	20 (11–28)	< 1 (< 0 –< 1)	4 (< 1–7)

Antiproliferative (CVS assay) and cytotoxic (MTS assay) effects of BBS and NVX-207 on primary ES cells (sRGO1 and sRGO2), primary EMM cells (eRGO1 and MelDuWi) and primary equine dermal fibroblasts (PriFi1 and PriFi2) after a treatment duration of 5, 24, 48 or 96 h. Data represent mean IC_{50} values (µmol/L) of 6–9 independent experiments with 95% confidence interval in parentheses. "-" = Quantity of cells affected was too low to calculate IC_{50} values with the software applied; "n.a." = data not available

https://doi.org/10.1371/journal.pone.0241448.t002

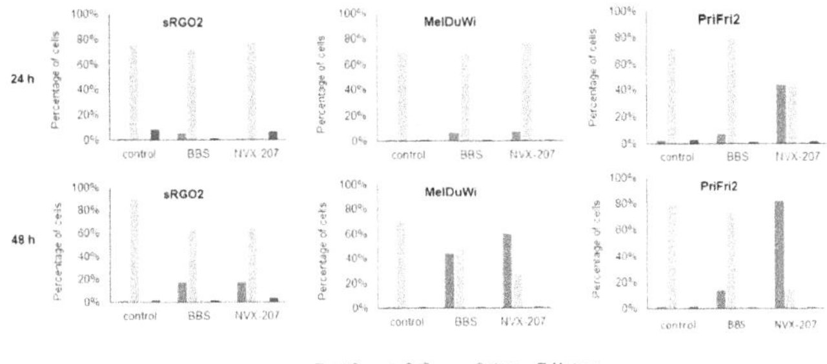

Fig 3. Cell cycle distributions of sRGO2, MelDuWi and PriFi2. Percentage of the four different phases in the cell cycle investigation of equine sarcoid (ES) cells (left), EMM cells (middle) and equine dermal fibroblasts (right) treated with BBS and NVX-207 at their double IC_{50} concentrations for 24 and 48 h. Magenta: subG1; light blue: G1/G0; grey: S-phase; and dark blue: G2/M-phase.

https://doi.org/10.1371/journal.pone.0241448.g003

cotton swabs and 32 ± 12% of the NVX-207 amount applied was detected in the skin. No NVX-207 was detected in the acceptor medium in any of the FDC experiments.

Discussion

The ES is the dermatologic neoplasm in equids diagnosed most frequently. The EMM is also a common skin tumor, especially in aging grey horses. In order to develop a topical therapy

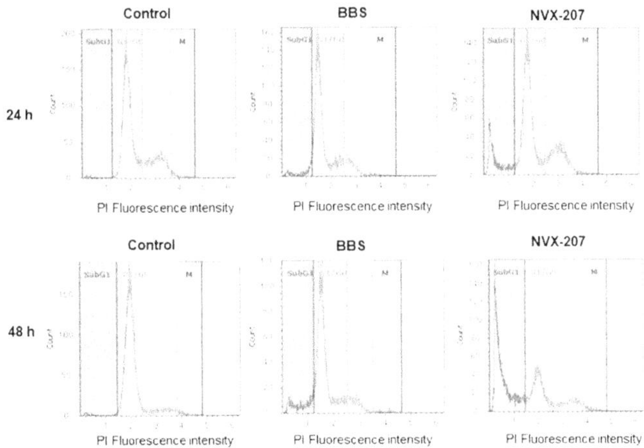

Fig 4. Cell cycle distributions for equine dermal fibroblasts PriFri2. The cells were untreated (control) or treated with BBS and NVX-207 at their double IC_{50} concentrations for 24 and 48 h (as indicated). The DNA was stained with propidium iodide and the cells were analyzed by flow cytometry. Red: SubG1 peak; light blue: G1/G0-phase peak; yellow: S-phase peak; and dark blue: G2/M-phase. (See S5–S10 Appendices for the interpretation of the other cell lines).

https://doi.org/10.1371/journal.pone.0241448.g004

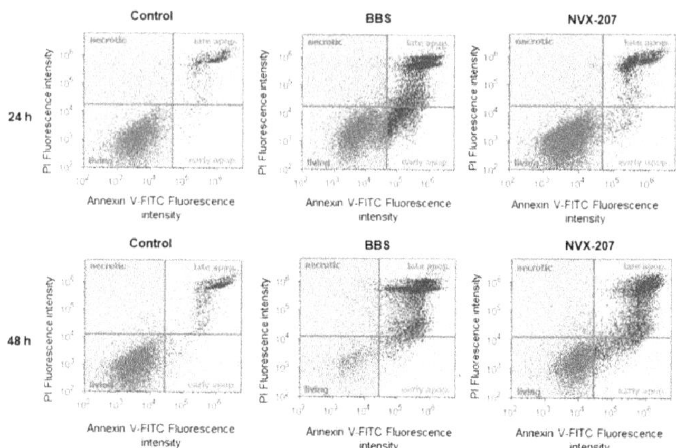

Fig 5. AnnexinV staining of ES cells sRGO2. The cells were untreated (control) or treated with BBS and NVX-207 at their double IC_{50} concentrations for 24 and 48 h (as indicated). After harvesting, the cells were stained and flow cytometry analysis was performed. Red: necrotic cells; green: late apoptotic cells; blue: early apoptotic cells; and magenta: living cells.

https://doi.org/10.1371/journal.pone.0241448.g005

against the ES and EMM, the betulinic acid derivative NVX-207 and the betulin derivative BBS were assessed for their antiproliferative, cytotoxic and apoptotic effects on ES cells, EMM cells and fibroblasts *in vitro*. Both substances had significant anticancer effects on the cells and induced apoptosis. NVX-207 was revealed to be the more potent substance. Therefore, this

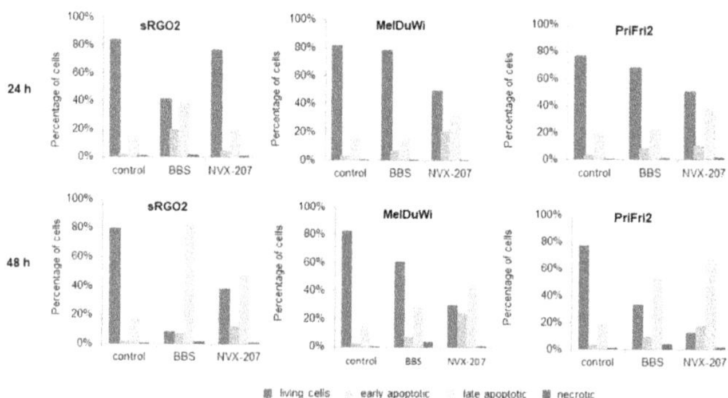

Fig 6. AnnexinV staining of equine cells. Equine sarcoid cells sRGO2, EMM cells MelDuWi and equine dermal fibroblasts PriFi2 were untreated (control) or treated with BBS and NVX-207 at their double IC_{50} concentrations for 24 and 48 h (as indicated) and used for the AnnexinV assay. Data shown are the percentages of living cells (magenta), early apoptotic cells (light blue), late apoptotic cells (green) and necrotic cells (red).

https://doi.org/10.1371/journal.pone.0241448.g006

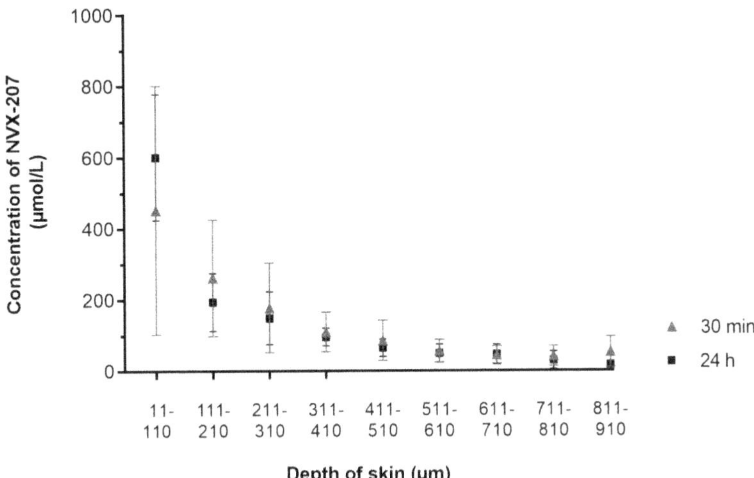

Fig 7. Concentration profile of NVX-207 correlative to skin thickness after 30 minutes and 24 hours of incubation. The skin of six horses (two technical replicates each) for each Franz-type diffusion cell experiment was used to investigate the permeation of 1% NVX-207 in "Basiscreme DAC" within 30 min and 24 h. The concentration of the compound for 30-min experiments was determined in 100 µm cryostat skin slices (pooled at 5 × 20 µm) at different skin depths by HPLC analysis. The 20-µm slices for 24-h experiments were stored and analyzed separately up to a depth of 310 µm. The slices were then pooled at 5 x 20 µm until a depth of a maximal of 910 µm was reached. All data are given per 100 µm skin depth in this figure for better comparison of the 30-min and 24-h concentration profiles. A more detailed version of the 24-h permeation profile is provided in the supplemented appendix (S21 Appendix). An incubation time of 24 h led to an accumulation of the compound in the upper epidermis (11–30 µm) but did not increase the amount of NVX-207 in the other skin layers analyzed. Figure data represent the mean concentration of NVX-207 at the skin depths indicated ± SD. Data for the 10-µm skin depth (*stratum corneum*) with potential test compound residues were excluded in this figure.

https://doi.org/10.1371/journal.pone.0241448.g007

compound was used for further *in vitro* permeation studies, where it was demonstrated that high concentrations could be reached in isolated equine skin.

The compound NVX-207 was previously assessed for its cytotoxic effects on EMM cells "MelDuWi" with the sulforhodamine B assay and a 96-h IC_{50} value of 5.6 µmol/L was reported [66]. Results of this first study on EMM cells "MelDuWi" could be replicated in the present study with different methodological approaches (CVS and MTS assay to assess the antiproliferative and cytotoxic effects, respectively) and widened by investigations with EMM cells "eRGO1," ES cells "sRGO1" and "sRGO2," and equine dermal fibroblasts "PriFi1" and "PriFi2." Three further treatment time points (5, 24 and 48 h) were included in the experiments to provide more information about the time-dependent efficacy of the drug. It was demonstrated that the antiproliferative and cytotoxic effects on ES cells, EMM cells and dermal fibroblasts enhanced with an increased treatment duration in a dose-dependent manner. After 48 and 96 h, very low concentrations of NVX-207 were sufficient to observe an inhibitory effect on the cells' proliferation and survival rate (e.g. for EMM cells eRGO1 < 1 µmol/L in CVS and MTS assay after 96 h of incubation). In addition, after 5 h of drug exposure, the quantity of affected cells was already high enough to calculate IC_{50} values, substantiating the potent effects of NVX-207 on equine cells. These data could be taken into account when prospective *in vivo* treatment regimens are designed.

This study is the first report on the influence of NVX-207 on ES cells and normal equine dermal fibroblasts. NVX-207 had cell viability reducing and antiproliferative effects on both cell types. The similar treatment response of the cells is not surprising, as the ES is addressed as a tumor of the fibroblasts [12]. However, compared to normal equine cells, a selectivity of the compound to ES cells could be demonstrated in the proliferation assay, suggesting that sarcoid cells are even more sensitive. A selectivity of NVX-207 to EMM cells was not observed. The same was shown for EMM cells and fibroblasts when treated with the parent BA [45]. In contrast to these findings, it was reported that NVX-207 had little impact on the *in vitro* survival of normal human umbilical vein endothelial cells, fibroblasts and keratinocytes [64]. Furthermore, current *in vivo* data indicate a good systemic and local tolerability of 1% NVX-207 after topical application twice a day for seven consecutive days in eight healthy horses [67]. In addition, the intralesional injection of the compound in two EMM patients once a week for 19 consecutive weeks proved to be safe [66]. Intravenous application of the compound in mice did not lead to any side effects [64] and the intralesional treatment of different malignancies in five dogs was well tolerated and clinically beneficial tumor response was observed [64].

It has been demonstrated previously that NVX-207 triggers the mitochondrial-induced apoptotic pathway in human melanoma cell lines via activation of caspases-9, -3 and -7 and cleavage of poly (ADP-ribose) polymerase [64]. Furthermore, an increase of subG1 cells after treatment of various human cancer cell lines with BA and NVX-207 has been reported [72, 73]. An induction of both initiator caspases (caspase-8 and caspase-9) in EMM cells led to an activation of effector caspase-3 [66]. Comparable to a treatment with the parent BA, an accumulation of EMM cells in the subG1 phase and externalization of phosphatidylserines to the extracellular side of the plasma membrane, a characteristic feature of apoptosis, were observed after treatment with NVX-207 [66]. These preliminary investigations by Liebscher et al. on EMM cells MelDuWi could be reproduced in this study. However, up to now, no data on the molecular mechanisms in ES cells and normal equine cells after treatment with NVX-207 has existed. Cell cycle investigations and AnnexinV staining were performed to address this lack. Results from these apoptosis tests demonstrated that NVX-207 triggers apoptosis in ES cells sRGO2. However, the effects were less pronounced compared to EMM cells MelDuWi and equine dermal fibroblasts PriFi2. After 48 h, the number of apoptotic cells detected with AnnexinV staining was about 60%, of which 48% were late apoptotic. Only 17% of the cells were found to be in the subG1 phase with a fragmented DNA. The different quantity of apoptotic cells analyzed with different methods may be explained by the temporally staggered occurrence of characteristic cellular changes, which are made visible by the respective method. The results reported here further indicate that similar modes of action observed in equine cancer cells also take place in unaltered equine cells when treated with NVX-207. After an incubation of 48 h, about 85% of equine dermal fibroblasts PriFi2 were apoptotic and a clear shift to cells in the subG1 phase was already observed after 24 h of treatment. It is remarkable that the proportion of necrotic cells, whether in altered or normal cell types, was below 2% after a treatment of 48 h. Even though the results reported from *in vitro* experiments with equine skin cancer cells are promising, it must be emphasized that cells in their native microenvironment can be much more robust against (phyto)chemotherapeutic influences [74–76]. Therefore, no reliable conclusions can be drawn regarding the efficacy of a topical NVX-207 application in ES and EMM patients and prospective *in vivo* studies have made to address this question.

The betulin derivative BBS had significant antiproliferative and cytotoxic effects on all three cell types investigated in the present study, however, it was considerably less effective compared to NVX-207. In addition, the IC_{50} values of BBS calculated for EMM cells were higher than the ones reported for BA [45, 66]. Therefore, further permeation studies were performed with NVX-207. Nevertheless, in contrast to NVX-207, the compound was less toxic for normal cells. In order to clarify the cellular pathways of BBS in ES cells, EMM cells and equine dermal fibroblasts, it was shown by AnnexinV staining and cell cycle investigations that BBS induced apoptosis in these cells. However, while the apoptotic impact of BBS was stronger in sarcoid cells compared to the effects of NVX-207 in these equine skin cancer cells, this was not the case for EMM cells and fibroblasts. In EMM cells, the amount of late apoptotic cells after 48 h was 44.8% (NVX-207) compared to 28.2% (BBS). Regarding the results from the proliferation test and the cell cycle analysis, there seems to be a selectivity of BBS towards equine skin cancer cells in comparison to unaltered equine dermal fibroblasts. In addition, AnnexinV staining revealed a preferred triggering of the programmed cell death for the sarcoid cells (82.1% late apoptotic after a 48-h treatment with BBS) when compared to the late apoptotic phase of fibroblasts (53.6%). However, only 28.2% of EMM cells were late apoptotic at this stage.

In addition to its apoptotic effects, it should be noted that BBS has been demonstrated to be an efficient inhibitor of human carbonic anhydrase isoenzymes I, II and IX [63]. Carbonic anhydrase IX is overexpressed in many tumors and involved in complex pathways leading to changes in the tumor microenvironment and subsequent tumor progression [77]. Human malignant melanoma cells also express this enzyme and a combination of proton pump and carbonic anhydrase IX inhibitors led to enhanced anticancer effects in these cells *in vitro* [78]. Further investigations are necessary to confirm and expand these results in equine malignancies, however, carbonic anhydrase inhibitors such as BBS could represent potential candidates as anti-tumor agents alone or adjunctive therapeutic drugs.

Except for ulcerated tumors, histopathologic examinations address the localization of melanocytic skin tumors in horses mostly as "dermal" or "subcutaneous" [79, 80]. The ES is regarded as a neoplasm of the dermal fibroblasts, which appear with an increased density and proliferation [81, 82]. Epidermal alterations, such as hyperplasia, hyperkeratosis or rete pig formation, vary between the different clinical ES types but are present in the majority of cases [82]. Due to the tumors' microscopic appearance, the topically applied compound NVX-207 needs to liberate from the drug formulation, penetrate the body protective *stratum corneum* and permeate through the viable epidermal and dermal strata to reach the sarcoid and melanoma cells. A standardized use of ES or EMM skin was not possible for FDC experiments due to technical reasons, which is a limitation of the study. Therefore, normal thoracic equine skin was utilized, as described previously [45, 83].

It has been reported previously that high concentrations of BA could be reached in isolated equine skin when 1% of the compound was mixed in "Basiscreme DAC" with 20% medium-chain triglycerides [45]. Therefore, a drug formulation containing "Basiscreme DAC" with 20% medium-chain triglycerides and 1% of betulinic acid derivative NVX-207 (test formulation 1) was initially tested for *in vitro* permeation. A significant phase separation was already observed 24 h after the production of test formulation 1. The oily sediments were probably the 20% medium-chain triglycerides added, which coalesced as the emulsifier system combined with 1% NVX-207 was presumably not strong enough to form a stable emulsion with the additional fatty acids. The inhomogeneous distribution of NVX-207 suspected in test formulation 1 was confirmed when less than 50% of the substance, which had allegedly been applied on the diffusion area, was detected in the HPLC analysis. The drug formulation was improved as such a low recovery rate in permeation studies and such high variations of active compound distribution in the cream are not acceptable for a topical medication. When 1% NVX-207 was mixed with "Basiscreme DAC" but without additional medium-chain triglycerides (test formulation 2), no phase separation was observed by visual inspection and the overall recovery rate was above 85%.

There was a nearly identical concentration profile of the compound in isolated equine skin when incubated for 30 min and 24 h, except for a considerable difference in the upper epidermal layers. This indicates a rapid penetration of the lipophilic NVX-207 through the *stratum corneum* and accumulation in the viable epidermal skin layers, followed by a slower permeation into the subjacent, more hydrophilic dermal skin layers [84, 85]. As the blood circulation in *in vitro* FDC experiments is missing, no compound is absorbed by dermal capillary blood vessels, which could further explain the steady state between the 30-min and 24-h permeation studies. Regarding the *in vitro* data determined about antiproliferative and cytotoxic effects of NVX-207 towards ES cells and EMM cells reported here and formerly for EMM cells [66], the concentrations of the compound reached up to a depth of 810 μm in isolated equine skin after 30 min and 24 h of incubation *in vitro* would be sufficient to have an inhibitory or even cytotoxic impact on the cells' metabolism. This might suggest that the proliferation and survival rate of ES and EMM cells especially in the superficial dermal skin layer could be reduced by NVX-207 *in vivo*. However, as mentioned previously, the epidermal nature in ES varies and epidermal thickening can influence the permeation rate of a topically applied drug negatively [86]. Furthermore, it should be considered that the *in vitro* permeation of acyclovir in ES skin differs significantly from epidermal to superficial dermal and deep dermal skin layers and that less acyclovir was found in the deep dermal layers of sarcoid skin compared to normal skin [87]. By contrast, the *in vitro* concentration profiles of NVX-207 in thoracic skin and hairless EMM predilection site skin (e.g. undersurface on the tail, perianal region) can be assumed to be comparable, as the concentrations of hydrocortisone, a lipophilic substance similar to NVX-207, did not differ significantly in the clipped thoracic equine skin and nearly glabrous groin skin [88]. However, an increased vascularization was described in some EMM [31, 79]. Compound elimination by dermal blood vessels cannot be evaluated by FDC experiments and, therefore, the permeated dose required to exert antitumoral effects *in vivo* can also be significantly higher. Furthermore, an encapsulation of the tumor could reduce the drug permeation rate at the treatment site. Because the *in vitro* anticancer effects were demonstrated to be concentration- and time-dependent, prospective *in vivo* treatment regimens with short application intervals and long treatment durations could favorably influence the concentration and efficacy of NVX-207 in the skin of ES and EMM patients.

Conclusion

In conclusion, the betulinic acid derivative NVX-207 has a superior antiproliferative and cell viability reducing effect on primary ES cells and EMM cells compared to BBS. Both compounds induced apoptosis. High concentrations of NVX-207 were reached in isolated equine skin–even after only 30 min of incubation–demonstrating a potent skin permeation. Although the *in vitro* data reported are promising, the results are not unconditionally applicable to the clinical situation. Therefore, *in vivo* studies are needed to assess the antitumoral effects of topically applied NVX-207 in equine patients suffering from ES or EMM.

Supporting information

S1 Appendix. IC_{50} values measured by SRB Assay after 96 h. IC_{50} values (μmol/L) of betulinyl-bis-sulfamate (BBS) and NVX-207 thereof on three equine cell types (equine sarcoid [ES] cells sRGO2, equine malignant melanoma [EMM] cells MelDuWi and equine dermal fibroblasts PriFi2) determined by SRB-Assay after 96 h of drug exposure. Measurements were carried out at least as thrice determination.
(DOCX)

S2 Appendix. Cytotoxicity dose-response curves of BBS and NVX-207. ES cells sRGO2 (left), EMM (middle) and equine fibroblasts PriFri2 (right) determined by SRB Assay after 96

h (one representative of three independent experiments).
(PNG)

S3 Appendix. Effects of BBS and NVX-207 on primary equine cell proliferation at different time points. Proliferation dose-response regression lines of BBS and NVX-207 on primary ES cells (sRGO1, sRGO2) and primary equine dermal fibroblasts (PriFi1, PriFi2) at three different time points (5, 24 and 48 h) determined by crystal violet staining assay. Antiproliferative effects of the compounds on primary equine cells increase with concentration and time of drug exposition. Data represent regression lines and 95% confidence intervals of 6–8 independent experiments for each combination of cell type, incubation time and concentration. Concentrations at which the corresponding 95% confidence intervals do not cross the 100% line indicate a significant reduction of the proliferation rate.
(PNG)

S4 Appendix. Effects of BBS and NVX-207 on primary equine cell viability at different time points. Proliferation dose-response regression lines of BBS and NVX-207 on primary ES cells (sRGO1, sRGO2) and primary equine dermal fibroblasts (PriFi1, PriFi2) at three different time points (5, 24 and 48 h) determined by MTS assay. Cytotoxic effects of the compounds on primary equine cells increase with concentration and time of drug exposition. Data represent regression lines and 95% confidence intervals of 6–8 independent experiments for each combination of cell type, incubation time and concentration. Concentrations at which the corresponding 95% confidence intervals do not cross the 100% line indicate a significant reduction of the cell viability rate.
(PNG)

S5 Appendix. Cell cycle distributions of ES cells sRGO2. Cells were untreated (control) or treated with BBS and NVX-207 at their double IC_{50} concentrations for 24 and 48 h (as indicated). The DNA was stained with propidium iodide and the cells were analyzed by flow cytometry. Red: SubG1 peak; light blue: G1/G0 phase peak; Yellow: S-phase peak; and dark blue: G2/M phase.
(PNG)

S6 Appendix. Cell cycle percentage of ES cells sRGO2. Cells were untreated (control) or treated with BBS and NVX-207 at their double IC_{50} concentrations for 24 h.
(DOCX)

S7 Appendix. Cell cycle percentage of ES cells sRGO2. Cell were untreated (control) or treated with BBS and NVX-207 at their double IC_{50} concentrations for 48 h.
(DOCX)

S8 Appendix. Cell cycle distributions of EMM cells MelDuWi. Cells were untreated (control) or treated with BBS and NVX-207 at their double IC_{50} concentrations for 24 and 48 h (as indicated). The DNA was stained with propidium iodide and the cells were analyzed by flow cytometry. Red: SubG1 peak; light blue: G1/G0 phase peak; Yellow: S-phase peak; and dark blue: G2/M phase.
(PNG)

S9 Appendix. Cell cycle percentage of EMM MelDuWi. Cells were untreated (control) or treated with BBS and NVX-207 at their double IC_{50} concentrations for 24 h.
(DOCX)

S10 Appendix. Cell cycle percentage of EMM MelDuWi. Cells were untreated (control) or treated with BBS and NVX-207 at their double IC_{50} concentrations for 48 h.
(DOCX)

S11 Appendix. Cell cycle percentage of equine dermal fibroblasts PriFri2. Cells were untreated (control) or treated with BBS and NVX-207 at their double IC_{50} concentrations for 24 h.
(DOCX)

S12 Appendix. Cell cycle percentage of equine dermal fibroblasts PriFri2. Cells were untreated (control) or treated with BBS and NVX-207 at their double IC_{50} concentrations for 48 h.
(DOCX)

S13 Appendix. AnnexinV staining. Percentage of ES cells sRGO2 untreated (control) or treated with BBS and NVX-207 at their double IC_{50} concentrations for 24 h.
(DOCX)

S14 Appendix. AnnexinV staining. Percentage of ES cells sRGO2 untreated (control) or treated with BBS and NVX-207 at their double IC_{50} concentrations for 48 h.
(DOCX)

S15 Appendix. AnnexinV staining of equine dermal fibroblasts PriFri2. Cells were untreated (control) or treated with BBS and NVX-207 at their double IC_{50} concentrations for 24 and 48 h (as indicated). After harvesting, the cells were stained and flow cytometry analysis was performed. Red: necrotic cells; green: late apoptotic cells; blue: early apoptotic cells; magenta: living cells.
(PNG)

S16 Appendix. AnnexinV staining. Percentage of equine dermal fibroblasts PriFri2 untreated (control) or treated with BBS and NVX-207 at their double IC_{50} concentrations for 24 h.
(DOCX)

S17 Appendix. AnnexinV staining. Percentage of equine dermal fibroblasts PriFri2 untreated (control) or treated with BBS and NVX-207 at their double IC_{50} concentrations for 48 h.
(DOCX)

S18 Appendix. AnnexinV staining of EMM cells MelDuWi. Cells were untreated (control) or treated with BBS and NVX-207 at their double IC50 concentrations for 24 and 48 h (as indicated). After harvesting, the cells were stained and flow cytometry analysis was performed. Red: necrotic cells; green: late apoptotic cells; blue: early apoptotic cells; magenta: living cells.
(PNG)

S19 Appendix. AnnexinV staining. Percentage of EMM cells (MelDuWi) untreated (control) or treated with BBS and NVX-207 at their double IC_{50} concentrations for 24 h.
(DOCX)

S20 Appendix. AnnexinV staining. Percentage of EMM cells (MelDuWi) untreated (control) or treated with BBS and NVX-207 at their double IC_{50} concentrations for 48 h.
(DOCX)

S21 Appendix. Concentration profile of NVX-207 correlative to skin thickness after 24 h of incubation. The skin of six horses (two technical replicates each) were used to investigate the permeation of 1% NVX-207 in "Basiscreme DAC" within 24 h for the Franz-type diffusion cell experiment. The concentration of the compound was determined in 20 μm and 100 μm (deeper skin layers; pooled at 5 × 20 μm) cryostat skin slices at different skin depths by HPLC analysis. Figure data represent mean concentration of NVX-207 at the skin depth indicated and ± SD. Data for 10-μm skin depth (*stratum corneum*) with potential test compound

residues were excluded from this figure.
(TIF)

Acknowledgments

The authors thank Dr. Barbara Pratscher and Dr. Sabine Brandt, both Research Group Oncology, University Equine Clinic, University of Veterinary Medicine Vienna, Vienna, Austria, for providing EMM cells "eRGO1" and ES cells "sRGO1" and "sRGO2", respectively. The authors thank the Department of Pathology, University of Veterinary Medicine Hannover Foundation, Hannover, for providing equine thoracic skin for the FDC experiments. The authors thank Dr. Konstanze Bosse, Skinomics GmbH, Halle, Germany for good advice regarding questions regarding the pharmaceutical test formulations.

Author Contributions

Conceptualization: Reinhard Paschke, Jessica Meißner, Manfred Kietzmann, Jessika-Maximiliane V. Cavalleri.

Formal analysis: Lisa Annabel Weber, Anne Funtan, Julien Delarocque.

Funding acquisition: Reinhard Paschke, Karsten Feige, Jessika-Maximiliane V. Cavalleri.

Investigation: Lisa Annabel Weber, Anne Funtan, Jutta Kalbitz.

Methodology: Jutta Kalbitz.

Project administration: Lisa Annabel Weber, Reinhard Paschke, Jessika-Maximiliane V. Cavalleri.

Supervision: Reinhard Paschke, Jessica Meißner, Karsten Feige, Manfred Kietzmann, Jessika-Maximiliane V. Cavalleri.

Visualization: Lisa Annabel Weber, Anne Funtan, Julien Delarocque.

Writing – original draft: Lisa Annabel Weber.

Writing – review & editing: Lisa Annabel Weber, Anne Funtan, Reinhard Paschke, Manfred Kietzmann.

References

1. Scott DW, Miller WH. Equine dermatology. 2nd ed. Maryland Heights: Elsevier Saunders; 2011.
2. Scott D, Miller W. Equine dermatology I. S. Louis; 2003.
3. Valentine B. Survey of equine cutaneous neoplasia in the Pacific Northwest. J Vet Diagnostic Investig. 2006; 18:123–126. https://doi.org/10.1177/104063870601800121 PMID: 16566271
4. Goodrich L, Gerber H, Marti E, Antczak DF. Equine sarcoids. Vet Clin North Am Equine Pract. 1998; 14:607–623. https://doi.org/10.1016/S0749-0739(17)30189-X PMID: 9891727
5. Pascoe RR, Summers PM. Clinical survey of tumours and tumour-like lesions in horses in south east Queensland. Equine Vet J. 1981; 13:235–239. https://doi.org/10.1111/j.2042-3306.1981.tb03504.x PMID: 6459231
6. Baker JR, Leyland A. Histological survey of tumours of the horse, with particular reference to those of the skin. Vet Rec. 1975; 96:419–422. https://doi.org/10.1136/vr.96.19.419 PMID: 1173477
7. Marti E, Lazary S, Antczak DF, Gerber H. Report of the first international workshop on equine sarcoid. Equine Vet J. 1993; 25:397–407. https://doi.org/10.1111/j.2042-3306.1993.tb02981.x PMID: 8223371
8. Chambers G, Ellsmore VA, O'Brien PM, Reid SWJ, Love S, Campo MS, et al. Association of bovine papillomavirus with the equine sarcoid. J Gen Virol. 2003; 84:1055–1062. https://doi.org/10.1099/vir.0.18947-0 PMID: 12692268

9. Yuan ZQ, Gault EA, Saveria Campo M, Nasir L. Different contribution of bovine papillomavirus type 1 oncoproteins to the transformation of equine fibroblasts. J Gen Virol. 2011; 92:773–783. https://doi.org/10.1099/vir.0.028191-0 PMID: 21177927

10. Martens A, De Moor A, Ducatelle R. PCR detection of bovine papilloma virus DNA in superficial swabs and scrapings from equine sarcoids. Vet J. 2001; 161:280–286. https://doi.org/10.1053/tvjl.2000.0524 PMID: 11352485

11. Hainisch EK, Brandt S. Equine Sarcoid. Seventh Ed. Elsevier Inc.; 2014. https://doi.org/10.1016/B978-1-4557-4555-5.00099-6 PMID: 24467610

12. Knottenbelt DC. A suggested clinical classification for the equine sarcoid. Clin Tech Equine Pract. 2005; 4:278–295. https://doi.org/10.1053/j.ctep.2005.10.008.

13. Staiger EA, Tseng CT, Miller D, Cassano JM, Nasir L, Garrick D, et al. Host genetic influence on papillomavirus-induced tumors in the horse. Int J Cancer. 2016; 139:784–792. https://doi.org/10.1002/ijc.30120 PMID: 27037728

14. Angelos J, Oppenheim Y, Rebhun W, Mohammed H, Antczak DF. Evaluation of breed as a risk factor for sarcoid and uveitis in horses. Anim Genet. 1988; 19:417–425. https://doi.org/10.1111/j.1365-2052.1988.tb00833.x PMID: 3232865

15. Knottenbelt DC. The equine sarcoid: why are there so many treatment options? Vet Clin North Am—Equine Pract. 2019; 35:243–262. https://doi.org/10.1016/j.cveq.2019.03.006 PMID: 31097356

16. Stadler S, Kainzbauer C, Haralambus R, Brehm W, Hainisch E, Brandt S. Successful treatment of equine sarcoids by topical aciclovir application. Vet Rec. 2011; 168:1–4. https://doi.org/10.1136/vr.c5430 PMID: 21493530

17. Haspeslagh M, Jordana Garcia M, Vlaminck LEM, Martens AM. Topical use of 5% acyclovir cream for the treatment of occult and verrucous equine sarcoids: A double-blinded placebo-controlled study. BMC Vet Res. 2017; 13:1–6. https://doi.org/10.1186/s12917-017-1215-0 PMID: 28049469

18. Nogueira SAF, Torres SMF, Malone ED, Diaz SF, Jessen C, Gilbert S. Efficacy of imiquimod 5% cream in the treatment of equine sarcoids: A pilot study. Vet Dermatol. 2006; 17:259–265. https://doi.org/10.1111/j.1365-3164.2006.00526.x PMID: 16827669

19. Wilford S, Woodward E, Dunkel B. Owners' perception of the efficacy of Newmarket bloodroot ointment in treating equine sarcoids. Can Vet J. 2014; 55:683–686. PMID: 24982522

20. Taylor S, Haldorson G. A review of equine sarcoid. Equine Vet Educ. 2013; 25:210–216. https://doi.org/10.1111/j.2042-3292.2012.00411.x.

21. Teixeira RBC, Rendahl AK, Anderson SM, Mickelson JR, Sigler D, Buchanan BR, et al. Coat color genotypes and risk and severity of melanoma in gray quarter horses. J Vet Intern Med. 2013; 27:1201–1208. https://doi.org/10.1111/jvim.12133 PMID: 23875712

22. Seltenhammer MH, Simhofer H, Scherzer S, Zechner P, Curik I, Sölkner J, et al. Equine melanoma in a population of 296 grey Lipizzaner horses. Equine Vet J. 2003; 35:153–157. https://doi.org/10.2746/042516403776114234 PMID: 12638791

23. Fleury C, Bérard F, Balme B, Thomas L. The study of cutaneous melanomas in Camargue-type gray-skinned horses (1): clinical-pathological characterization. Pigment Cell Res. 2000; 13:39–46. https://doi.org/10.1034/j.1600-0749.2000.130108.x PMID: 10761995

24. McFadyean J. Equine melanomatosis. J Comp Pathol Ther. 1933; 46:186–204. http://dx.doi.org/10.1016/S0368-1742(33)80025-7.

25. Rodriguez M, Garcia-Barona V, Pena L, Castano M, Rodriguez A. Grey Horse Melanotic Condition: J Equine Vet Sci 1997; 17:677–81.

26. Valentine BA. Equine melanocytic tumors: a retrospective study of 53 horses (1988 to 1991). J Vet Intern Med. 1995; 9:291–297. https://doi.org/10.1111/j.1939-1676.1995.tb01087.x PMID: 8531173

27. Rosengren Pielberg G, Golovko A, Sundström E, Curik I, Lennartsson J, Seltenhammer MH, et al. A cis-acting regulatory mutation causes premature hair graying and susceptibility to melanoma in the horse. Nat Genet. 2008; 40:1004–1009. https://doi.org/10.1038/ng.185 PMID: 18641652

28. Sundström E, Komisarczuk AZ, Jiang L, Golovko A, Navratilova P, Rinkwitz S, et al. Identification of a melanocyte-specific, microphthalmia-associated transcription factor-dependent regulatory element in the intronic duplication causing hair greying and melanoma in horses. Pigment Cell Melanoma Res. 2012; 25:28–36. https://doi.org/10.1111/j.1755-148X.2011.00902.x PMID: 21883983

29. Macgillivray KC, Sweeney RW, Del Piero F. Metastatic melanoma in horses. J Vet Intern Med. 2002; 16:452–456.

30. Scott D. Neoplastic Diseases. In: Pedersen D, editor. Large animal dermatology. Philadelphia, USA: W.B. Saunders Company; 1988, p. 448–452.

31. Moore JS, Shaw C, Shaw E, Buechner-Maxwell V, Scarratt WK, Crisman M, et al. Melanoma in horses: current perspectives. Equine Vet Educ. 2013; 25:144–151. https://doi.org/10.1111/j.2042-3292.2011.00368.x.

32. Müller JMV, Feige K, Wunderlin P, Hödl A, Meli ML, Seltenhammer M, et al. Double-blind placebo-controlled study with interleukin-18 and interleukin-12-encoding plasmid DNA shows antitumor effect in metastatic melanoma in gray horses. J Immunother. 2011; 34:58–64. https://doi.org/10.1097/CJI.0b013e3181fe1997 PMID: 21150713

33. Phillips JC, Lembcke LM. Equine melanocytic tumors. Vet Clin North Am—Equine Pract. 2013; 29:673–687. https://doi.org/10.1016/j.cveq.2013.08.008 PMID: 24267683

34. Mählmann K, Feige K, Juhls C, Endmann A, Schuberth H-J, Oswald D, et al. Local and systemic effect of transfection-reagent formulated DNA vectors on equine melanoma. BMC Vet Res. 2015; 11:1–11. https://doi.org/10.1186/s12917-015-0422-9 PMID: 25582057

35. Laus F, Cerquetella M, Paggi E, Ippedico G, Argentieri M, Castellano G, et al. Evaluation of cimetidine as a therapy for dermal melanomatosis in grey horse. Isr J Vet Med. 2010; 65:47–52.

36. Goetz TE, Ogilvie GK, Keegan KG, Johnson PJ. Cimetidine for treatment of melanomas in three horses. J Am Vet Med Assoc. 1990; 196:449–452. PMID: 2298676

37. Bradley WM, Schilpp D, Khatibzadeh SM. Electronic brachytherapy used for the successful treatment of three different types of equine tumours. Equine Vet Educ. 2017; 29:293–298. https://doi.org/10.1111/eve.12420.

38. Groom LM, Sullins KE. Surgical excision of large melanocytic tumours in grey horses: 38 cases (2001–2013). Equine Vet Educ. 2018; 30:438–443. https://doi.org/10.1111/eve.12767.

39. Rowe EL, Sullins KE. Excision as treatment of dermal melanomatosis in horses: 11 cases (1994–2000). J Am Vet Med Assoc. 2004; 225:94–96. https://doi.org/10.2460/javma.2004.225.94 PMID: 15239480

40. Théon AP, Wilson WD, Magdesian KG, Pusterla N, Snyder JR, Galuppo LD. Long-term outcome associated with intratumoral chemotherapy with cisplatin for cutaneous tumors in equidae: 573 cases (1995–2004). J Am Vet Med Assoc. 2007; 230:1506–1513. https://doi.org/10.2460/javma.230.10.1506 PMID: 17504043

41. Hewes C, Sullins KE. Use of cisplatin-containing biodegradable beads for treatment of cutaneous neoplasia in equidae: 59 cases (2000–2004). J Am Vet Med Assoc. 2006; 229:1617–1622. https://doi.org/10.2460/javma.229.10.1617 PMID: 17107319

42. Scacco L, Bolaffio C, Romano A, Fanciulli M, Baldi A, Spugnini EP. Adjuvant electrochemotherapy increases local control in a recurring equine anal melanoma. J Equine Vet Sci. 2013; 33:637–639. https://doi.org/10.1016/j.jevs.2012.09.006.

43. Spugnini EP, D'Alterio GL, Dotsinsky I, Mudrov T, Dragonetti E, Murace R, et al. Electrochemotherapy for the treatment of multiple melanomas in a horse. J Equine Vet Sci. 2011; 31:430–433. https://doi.org/10.1016/j.jevs.2011.01.009.

44. Sanderson BJS, Ferguson LR, Denny WA. Mutagenic and carcinogenic properties of platinum-based anticancer drugs. Mutat Res—Fundam Mol Mech Mutagen. 1996; 355:59–70. https://doi.org/10.1016/0027-5107(96)00022-X PMID: 8781577

45. Weber LA, Meißner J, Delarocque J, Kalbitz J, Feige K, Kietzmann M, et al. Betulinic acid shows anticancer activity against equine melanoma cells and permeates isolated equine skin in vitro. BMC Vet Res. 2020; 16:1–9. https://doi.org/10.1186/s12917-020-2262-5 PMID: 31900161

46. Zalesińska MD, Borska S. Betulin and its derivatives–precursors of new drugs. World Sci News. 2019; 127:123–138.

47. Yogeeswari P, Sriram D. Betulinic acid and its derivatives: a review on their biological properties. Curr Med Chem. 2005; 12:657–666. https://doi.org/10.2174/0929867053202214 PMID: 15790304

48. Pisha E, Chai H, Lee I-S, Chagwedera TE, Farnsworth NHS, Cordell GA, et al. Discovery of betulinic acid as a selective inhibitor of human melanoma that functions by induction of apoptosis. Nat Med. 1995; 1:1046–1051. https://doi.org/10.1038/nm1095-1046 PMID: 7489361

49. Fulda S, Friesen C, Los M, Scaffidi C, Mier W, Benedict M, et al. Betulinic acid triggers CD95 (APO-1/Fas)- and p53-independent apoptosis via activation of caspases in neuroectodermal tumors. Cancer Res. 1997; 57:4956–4964. PMID: 9354463

50. Ali-Seyed M, Jantan I, Vijayaraghavan K, Bukhari SNA. Betulinic acid: recent advances in chemical modifications, effective delivery, and molecular mechanisms of a promising anticancer therapy. Chem Biol Drug Des. 2016; 87:517–536. https://doi.org/10.1111/cbdd.12682 PMID: 26535952

51. Ríos JL, Máñez S. New pharmacological opportunities for betulinic acid. Planta Med. 2018; 84:8–19. https://doi.org/10.1055/s-0043-123472 PMID: 29202513

52. Fulda S, Kroemer G. Targeting mitochondrial apoptosis by betulinic acid in human cancers. Drug Discov Today. 2009; 14:885–890. https://doi.org/10.1016/j.drudis.2009.05.015 PMID: 19520182

53. Fulda S, Scaffidi G, Susin SA, Krammer PH, Kroemer G, Peter ME, et al. Activation of mitochondria and release of mitochondrial apoptogenic factors by betulinic acid. J Biol Chem. 1998; 273:33942–33948. https://doi.org/10.1074/jbc.273.51.33942 PMID: 9852046

54. Mullauer FB, Kessler JH, Medema JP. Betulinic acid induces cytochrome c release and apoptosis in a Bax/Bak-independent, permeability transition pore dependent fashion. Apoptosis. 2009; 14:191–202. https://doi.org/10.1007/s10495-008-0290-x PMID: 19115109

55. Raghuvar Gopal D V., Narkar AA, Badrinath Y, Mishra KP, Joshi DS. Protection of Ewing's sarcoma family tumor (ESFT) cell line SK-N-MC from betulinic acid induced apoptosis by α-DL-tocopherol. Toxicol Lett. 2004; 153:201–212. https://doi.org/10.1016/j.toxlet.2004.03.027 PMID: 15451550

56. Tan YM, Yu R, Pezzuto JM. Betulinic acid-induced programmed cell death in human melanoma cells involves mitogen-activated protein kinase activation. Clin Cancer Res. 2003; 9:2866–2875. PMID: 12855667

57. Chowdhury RA, Mandal S, Mittra B, Sharma S, Mukhopadhyay S, Majumder HK. Betulinic acid, a potent inhibitor of eukaryotic topoisomerase I: identification of the inhibitory step, the major functional group responsible and development of more potent derivatives. Med Sci Monit. 2002; 8:254–260. PMID: 12118187

58. Gheorgheosu D, Jung M, Ören B, Schmid T, Dehelean C, Muntean D, et al. Betulinic acid suppresses NGAL-induced epithelial-to-mesenchymal transition in melanoma. Biol Chem. 2013; 394:773–781. https://doi.org/10.1515/hsz-2013-0106 PMID: 23399635

59. Karna E, Szoka L, Palka JA. Betulinic acid inhibits the expression of hypoxia-inducible factor 1α and vascular endothelial growth factor in human endometrial adenocarcinoma cells. Mol Cell Biochem. 2010; 340:15–20. https://doi.org/10.1007/s11010-010-0395-8 PMID: 20174965

60. Ren W, Qin L, Xu Y, Cheng N. Inhibition of betulinic acid to growth and angiogenesis of human colorectal cancer cell in nude mice. Chinese-German J Clin Oncol. 2010; 9:153–157. https://doi.org/10.1007/s10330-010-0002-1.

61. Gauthier C, Legault J, Lebrun M, Dufour P, Pichette A. Glycosidation of lupane-type triterpenoids as potent in vitro cytotoxic agents. Bioorganic Med Chem. 2006; 14:6713–6725. https://doi.org/10.1016/j.bmc.2006.05.075 PMID: 16787747

62. Csuk R. Betulinic acid and its derivatives: a patent review (2008–2013). Expert Opin Ther Pat. 2014; 24:913–923. https://doi.org/10.1517/13543776.2014.927441 PMID: 24909232

63. Winum JY, Pastorekova S, Jakubickova L, Montero JL, Scozzafava A, Pastorek J, et al. Carbonic anhydrase inhibitors: Synthesis and inhibition of cytosolic/tumor-associated carbonic anhydrase isozymes I, II, and IX with bis-sulfamates. Bioorganic Med Chem Lett. 2005; 15:579–584. https://doi.org/10.1016/j.bmcl.2004.11.058.

64. Willmann M, Wacheck V, Buckley J, Nagy K, Thalhammer J, Paschke R, et al. Characterization of NVX-207, a novel betulinic acid-derived anti-cancer compound. Eur J Clin Invest. 2009; 39:384–394. https://doi.org/10.1111/j.1365-2362.2009.02105.x PMID: 19309323

65. Bache M, Bernhardt S, Passin S, Wichmann H, Hein A, Zschornak M, et al. Betulinic acid derivatives NVX-207 and B10 for treatment of glioblastoma—an in vitro study of cytotoxicity and radiosensitization. Int J Mol Sci. 2014; 15:19777–19790. https://doi.org/10.3390/ijms151119777 PMID: 25361208

66. Liebscher G, Vanchangiri K, Mueller T, Feige K, Cavalleri JMV, Paschke R. In vitro anticancer activity of Betulinic acid and derivatives thereof on equine melanoma cell lines from grey horses and invivo safety assessment of the compound NVX-207 in two horses. Chem Biol Interact. 2016; 246:20–29. https://doi.org/10.1016/j.cbi.2016.01.002 PMID: 26772157

67. Weber LA, Puff C, Kalbitz J, Kietzmann M, Feige K, Bosse K, et al. Concentration profiles and safety of topically applied betulinic acid and NVX-207 in eight healthy horses—A randomized, blinded, placebo-controlled, crossover pilot study. J Vet Pharmacol Ther. 2020; 0:jvp.12903. https://doi.org/10.1111/jvp.12903 PMID: 32845519

68. Team RDC, R Development Core Team R. R: A Language and Environment for Statistical Computing. 2008. https://doi.org/10.1007/978-3-540-74686-7.

69. Wood SN. Fast stable restricted maximum likelihood and marginal likelihood estimation of semiparametric generalized linear models. J R Stat Soc Ser B Stat Methodol. 2011; 73:3–36. https://doi.org/10.1111/j.1467-9868.2010.00749.x.

70. Mourdjeva M, Kyurkchiev D, Mandinova A, Altankova I, Kehayov I, Kyurkchiev S. Dynamics of membrane translocation of phosphatidylserine during apoptosis detected by a monoclonal antibody. Apoptosis. 2005; 10:209–217. https://doi.org/10.1007/s10495-005-6076-5 PMID: 15711937

71. Fadok VA, Voelker DR, Campbell PA, Cohen JJ, Bratton DL, Henson PM. Exposure of phosphatidylserine on the surface of apoptotic lymphocytes triggers specific recognition and removal by macrophages. J Immunol. 1992; 148:2207–2216. PMID: 1545126

72. Kommera H, Kaluderović GN, Bette M, Kalbitz J, Fuchs P, Fulda S, et al. In vitro anticancer studies of α- and β-d-glucopyranose betulin anomers. Chem Biol Interact. 2010; 185:128–136. https://doi.org/10.1016/j.cbi.2010.02.038 PMID: 20193672

73. Kommera H, Kaluderović GN, Kalbitz J, Dräger B, Paschke R. Small structural changes of pentacyclic lupane type triterpenoid derivatives lead to significant differences in their anticancer properties. Eur J Med Chem. 2010; 45:3346–3353. https://doi.org/10.1016/j.ejmech.2010.04.018 PMID: 20472329

74. Ferreira D, Adega F, Chaves R. The importance of cancer cell lines as in vitro models in cancer methylome analysis and anticancer drugs testing. Oncogenomics cancer proteomics—Nov. approaches Biomarkers Discov. Ther. Targets Cancer, vol. 3, InTech; 2013, p. 139–166. https://doi.org/10.5772/53110.

75. Kapałczyńska M, Kolenda T, Przybyła W, Zajączkowska M, Teresiak A, Filas V, et al. 2D and 3D cell cultures–a comparison of different types of cancer cell cultures. Arch Med Sci. 2016; 14:910–919. https://doi.org/10.5114/aoms.2016.63743 PMID: 30002710

76. van Staveren WCG, Solís DYW, Hébrant A, Detours V, Dumont JE, Maenhaut C. Human cancer cell lines: Experimental models for cancer cells in situ? For cancer stem cells? Biochim Biophys Acta—Rev Cancer. 2009; 1795:92–103. https://doi.org/10.1016/j.bbcan.2008.12.004 PMID: 19167460

77. Supuran CT. Carbonic anhydrase inhibitors as emerging agents for the treatment and imaging of hypoxic tumors. Expert Opin Investig Drugs. 2018; 27:963–970. https://doi.org/10.1080/13543784.2018.1548608 PMID: 30426805

78. Federici C, Lugini L, Marino ML, Carta F, Iessi E, Azzarito T, et al. Lansoprazole and carbonic anhydrase IX inhibitors sinergize against human melanoma cells. J Enzyme Inhib Med Chem. 2016; 31:119–125. https://doi.org/10.1080/14756366.2016.1177525 PMID: 27142956

79. Seltenhammer MH, Heere-Ress E, Brandt S, Druml T, Jansen B, Pehamberger H, et al. Comparative histopathology of grey-horse-melanoma and human malignant melanoma. Pigment Cell Res. 2004; 17:674–681. https://doi.org/10.1111/j.1600-0749.2004.00192.x PMID: 15541026

80. Smith SH, Goldschmidt MH, McManus PM. A comparative review of melanocytic neoplasms. Vet Pathol. 2002; 39:651–678. https://doi.org/10.1354/vp.39-6-651 PMID: 12450197

81. Tarwid J, Fretz P, Clark E. Equine sarcoids: a study with emphasis on pathologic diagnosis. Compend Contin Educ Pract Vet. 1985; 7:293–301.

82. Martens A, De Moor A, Demeulemeester J, Ducatelle R. Histopathological characteristics of five clinical types of equine sarcoid. Res Vet Sci. 2000. https://doi.org/10.1053/rvsc.2000.0432 PMID: 11124103

83. Stahl J, Kietzmann M. The effects of chemical and physical penetration enhancers on the percutaneous permeation of lidocaine through equine skin. BMC Vet Res. 2014; 10:1–6. https://doi.org/10.1186/1746-6148-10-138 PMID: 24383544

84. Luís A, Ruela M, Perissinato AG, Esselin M, Lino DS. Evaluation of skin absorption of drugs from topical and transdermal formulations. Brazilian J Pharm Sci. 2016; 52:527–544. http://dx.doi.org/10.1590/S1984-82502016000300018.

85. Guy RH, Hadgraft J. Prediction of Drug Disposition Kinetics. J Pharm Sci. 1984, 73:883–87. https://doi.org/10.1002/jps.2600730706 PMID: 6470948

86. Prausnitz MR, Elias PM, Franz TJ, Schmuth M, Tsai J-C, Menon GK, et al. Skin barrier and transdermal drug delivery. Med Ther. 2012; 5:2065–2073.

87. Haspeslagh M, Taevernier L, Maes AA, Vlaminck LEM, De Spiegeleer B, Croubels SM, et al. Topical distribution of acyclovir in normal equine skin and equine sarcoids: An in vitro study. Res Vet Sci. 2016; 106:107–111. https://doi.org/10.1016/j.rvsc.2016.03.021 PMID: 27234546

88. Mills PC, Cross SE. Regional differences in the in vitro penetration of hydrocortisone through equine skin. J Vet Pharmacol Ther. 2006; 29:25–30. https://doi.org/10.1016/j.rvsc.2006.07.015 PMID: 16420298

4. Manuscript III:

Concentration profiles and safety of topically applied betulinic acid and NVX-207 in eight healthy horses – A randomized, blinded, placebo-controlled, crossover pilot study

Lisa A. Weber[1*], Christina Puff[2], Jutta Kalbitz[3], Manfred Kietzmann[4], Karsten Feige[1], Konstanze Bosse[5], Karl Rohn[6], Jessika-M.V. Cavalleri[7]

[1] Clinic for Horses, University of Veterinary Medicine Hannover, Foundation, Bünteweg 9, 30559 Hannover, Germany

[2] Department of Pathology, University of Veterinary Medicine Hannover, Foundation, Bünteweg 17, 30559 Hannover, Germany

[3] Biosolutions Halle GmbH, Weinbergweg 22, 06120 Halle (Saale), Germany

[4] Department of Pharmacology, Toxicology and Pharmacy, University of Veterinary Medicine Hannover, Foundation, Bünteweg 17, 30559 Hannover, Germany

[5] Skinomics GmbH, Weinbergweg 23, 06120 Halle (Saale), Germany

[6] Department of Biometry, Epidemiology and Information Processing, University of Veterinary Medicine Hannover, Foundation, Bünteweg 2, 30559, Hannover, Germany

[7] University Equine Clinic, University of Veterinary Medicine Vienna, Veterinärplatz 1, 1210 Vienna, Austria

[*] Corresponding author

Journal of Veterinary Pharmacology and Therapeutics 2020;00:1-11

Accepted: 28 July 2020, published online: 26 August 2020

DOI: 10.1111/JVP.12903

Contribution to the manuscript:

LAW contributed to the study design and data analysis, performed animal experiments and skin sample processing for HPLC analysis and drafted and edited the manuscript. CP performed the histopathologic analysis of the skin biopsies. JK developed and performed the HPLC analysis. MK contributed to the study design and aided in data analysis and manuscript editing. KF contributed to the study design and aided in data analysis. KB prepared test formulations and aided in data analysis. KR performed the statistical analysis of the data. JMVC contributed to the study design, data analysis and aided in the manuscript editing. All authors read and approved the final manuscript.

Received: 8 May 2020 | Revised: 28 July 2020 | Accepted: 28 July 2020

DOI: 10.1111/jvp.12903

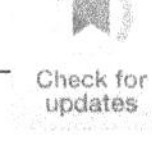

ORIGINAL ARTICLE

JOURNAL OF Veterinary Pharmacology and Therapeutics WILEY

Concentration profiles and safety of topically applied betulinic acid and NVX-207 in eight healthy horses—A randomized, blinded, placebo-controlled, crossover pilot study

Lisa A. Weber[1] | Christina Puff[2] | Jutta Kalbitz[3] | Manfred Kietzmann[4] | Karsten Feige[1] | Konstanze Bosse[5] | Karl Rohn[6] | Jessika-M. V. Cavalleri[7]

[1]Clinic for Horses, University of Veterinary Medicine Hannover, Foundation, Hannover, Germany

[2]Department of Pathology, University of Veterinary Medicine Hannover, Foundation, Hannover, Germany

[3]Biosolutions Halle GmbH, Halle (Saale), Germany

[4]Department of Pharmacology, Toxicology and Pharmacy, University of Veterinary Medicine Hannover, Foundation, Hannover, Germany

[5]Skinomics GmbH, Halle (Saale), Germany

[6]Department of Biometry, Epidemiology and Information Processing, University of Veterinary Medicine Hannover, Foundation, Hannover, Germany

[7]University Equine Clinic, University of Veterinary Medicine Vienna, Vienna, Austria

Correspondence
Lisa A. Weber, Clinic for Horses, University of Veterinary Medicine Hannover, Foundation, Bünteweg 9, 30559 Hannover, Germany.
Email: lisa.annabel.weber@tiho-hannover.de

Funding information
Bundesministerium für Wirtschaft und Energie, Grant/Award Number: 16KN051526, Open access funding enabled and organized by Projekt DEAL.

Abstract

The naturally occurring betulinic acid (BA) and its derivative NVX-207 show anti-cancer effects against equine malignant melanoma (EMM) cells and a potent permeation in isolated equine skin in vitro. The aim of the study was to determine the in vivo concentration profiles of BA and NVX-207 in equine skin and assess the compounds' local and systemic tolerability with the intent of developing a topical therapy against EMM. Eight horses were treated percutaneously in a crossover design with 1% BA, 1% NVX-207 or a placebo in a respective vehicle twice a day for seven consecutive days with a seven-day washout period between each formulation. Horses were treated at the neck and underneath the tail. Concentration profiles of the compounds were assessed by high-performance liquid chromatography in the cervical skin. Clinical and histopathological examinations and blood analyses were performed. Higher concentrations of NVX-207 were found in the skin compared to BA. Good systemic tolerability and only mild local adverse effects were observed in all three groups. This study substantiates the topical application of BA and NVX-207 in further clinical trials with horses suffering from EMM; however, penetration and permeation of the compounds may be altered in skin affected by tumors.

1 | INTRODUCTION

Dermatologic disorders are a common problem in horses (Scott & Miller, 2011; Traub-Dargatz, Salman, & Voss, 1991). Cutaneous neoplasms account for about 50% of all equine neoplasms (Baker & Leyland, 1975), and it has been reported that equine sarcoids, squamous cell carcinomas, papillomas, and melanomas are the skin cancers most frequently diagnosed in horses (Baker & Leyland, 1975; Scott & Miller, 2011; Valentine, 2006). The equine malignant melanoma (EMM) occurs primarily in gray horses and develops from the malignant transformation of normal melanocytes (Reed, Bayly, & Sellon, 2018; Smith, Goldschmidt, & McManus, 2002). The onset of the disease is usually characterized by the growth of small, solitary, raised tumors at glabrous predilection sites, such as the undersurface of the tail, perianal and perineal region, external genitalia, eyelids, and lips (Fleury, Bérard, Balme, & Thomas, 2000; Moore et al., 2013; Seltenhammer et al., 2010). Multiple and rapidly growing melanomas, which are capable of metastasizing, can occur with disease progression (Macgillivray, Sweeney, & Piero, 2002; Moore et al., 2013; Valentine, 1995). The EMM may reduce the horse's value and lead to economic losses due to cosmetic issues, interference with bit and bridle, and breeding impairment (Johnson, 1998; Sutton & Coleman, 1997). However, even more severe clinical problems, such as tumor ulceration with secondary bacterial infection, fecal impaction, osteomyelitis, and signs arising from lymphatic and hematogenous visceral metastasis, have been reported (Macgillivray et al., 2002; Moore et al., 2013; Patterson-Kane, Sanchez, Uhl, & Edens, 2001; Rodríguez, Forga, Herráez, Andrada, & Fernández, 1998; Smith et al., 2002). The few systemic and local therapies described for EMM are of varying efficacy (MacKay, 2019; Moore et al., 2013; Phillips & Lembcke, 2013). Commercially available, validated topical (epicutaneous) treatment options for this skin cancer are currently missing. One study describes the topical use of the triphenylethylene derivative toremifene in a horse affected by melanoma, which resulted in a slight volume reduction of the neoplasm (Soe et al., 1997). Positive therapeutic effects after topical application of frankincense oil in five EMM horses are reported in a PhD thesis (Moore, 2013). However, results from both studies were never confirmed in further evidence-based clinical trials.

The advantages of topical therapies for skin tumors include the noninvasiveness of the treatment and the possibility of comfortable drug application even on unfavorable treatment sites (Nogueira et al., 2006). Furthermore, the treatment can be conducted easily by the horse owners without the need for specialized equipment or facilities. Finally, undesired systemic side effects can be reduced (Luís, Ruela, Perissinato, Esselin, & Lino, 2016).

The naturally occurring betulinic acid (BA) and synthetically modified BA derivative NVX-207 have been demonstrated to exert antiproliferative and cytotoxic effects in equine melanoma cells in vitro, which is mediated by the induction of apoptosis (Liebscher et al., 2016; Weber, Meißner, et al., 2020; Weber, Funtan, et al., 2020, under review). Furthermore, a sufficient penetration and permeation of both compounds in isolated equine skin has been reported, as assessed by Franz-type diffusion cell (FDC) experiments (Weber, Meißner, et al., 2020; Weber, Funtan, et al., 2020, under review). After application of 1% formulations, the in vitro concentration profiles determined in the integument exceeded the half-maximal inhibitory concentrations (IC_{50}) for equine melanoma cells in the epidermal layers and superficial and partially deep dermal skin layers (Weber, Meißner, et al., 2020; Weber, Funtan, et al., 2020, under review). Both methods, cell culture experiments and FDC studies, are valuable tools for the evaluation of the in vitro efficacy and quality of topical formulations. However, the whole complexity of a biological system, including the metabolism, distribution, and elimination of a therapeutic agent, cannot be reproduced by FDC experiments, and in vivo data may have to follow the initial evaluations (Luís et al., 2016; OECD, 2004; OECD/OCDE, 2004). Furthermore, as normal equine dermal fibroblasts are also sensitive toward BA and NVX-207 in vitro, it has been indicated that time- and concentration-dependent antiproliferative and cytotoxic effects cannot be ruled out for this cell type in vivo (Weber, Meißner, et al., 2020; Weber, Funtan, et al., 2020, under review). To the best of the authors' knowledge, no further literature exists about the effects of either compound on equine keratinocytes or other unaltered equine skin cells but fibroblasts. Apoptosis-like effects have been observed in normal human melanocytes after in vitro treatment with BA (Galgon, Wohlrab, & Dräger, 2005; Selzer et al., 2000). Normal human epithelial keratinocytes and immortalized keratinocytes reacted by enhanced differentiation and apoptosis, respectively (Galgon et al., 2005). Unfortunately, study results from clinical trials in humans evaluating the safety and efficacy of topical BA against dysplastic melanocytic nevus and cutaneous metastatic melanoma have never been published (Fulda, 2008; Zalesińska & Borska, 2019). The BA-derivative NVX-207 had little impact on the cell survival of normal human fibroblasts and keratinocytes in vitro (Willmann et al., 2009). When NVX-207 was injected intralesionally in canine and two equine tumor patients, it was well tolerated and only mild local adverse effects were observed in dogs (Liebscher et al., 2016; Willmann et al., 2009). However, so far, no data about the in vivo percutaneous permeation and safety of epicutaneously administered BA or NVX-207 have been reported in horses. In order to develop a topical therapy against EMM, the first objective of this pilot study was to assess the in vivo concentration profiles of BA and NVX-207 in equine skin when applied topically twice a day for seven consecutive days in eight healthy horses. The second objective was to evaluate the local and systemic tolerability of both compounds after epicutaneous application.

2 | MATERIAL AND METHODS

2.1 | Horses

The pilot permeation and safety studies were performed between May and September 2019 at the Clinic for Horses of the University of Veterinary Medicine Hannover, Foundation, Hannover, Germany. Animal experiments were approved by an animal welfare officer of the University of Veterinary Medicine Hannover, Foundation, and the State Office for Consumer Protection and Food Safety (LAVES) in accordance with the German Animal Welfare Law (LAVES Reference number: 18/2941). The VICH Guideline 43 "Target Animal Safety For Veterinary Pharmaceutical Products" (VICH, 2008) was followed regarding the experimental design (number of animals used for the study, clinical local and systemic examinations, histopathological examinations of skin biopsies). Eight horses (five mares, two geldings, and one stallion) with a median age of 14.5 years (range 7–23 years) and a median body weight of 587.5 kg (range 488–649 kg) were used for target animal safety and permeation studies. Coat colors included bay (3), black (2), chestnut (2), and gray (1). Apart from horse 7 and 8, all were long-term residents of the Clinic for Horses, University of Veterinary Medicine Hannover, Foundation. The horses, except for the stallion, were maintained outdoors on grass pastures before commencing the study. They were stabled during treatment periods but lunged or walked daily. They were fed with hay (2 kg/100 kg bodyweight) and a mix of pellets and muesli (1.5–2 kg/horse/day). Access to water was ad libitum.

2.2 | Topical treatment

The horses were topically treated with test formulations that had been previously tested in permeation studies with isolated equine skin (Weber, Meißner, et al., 2020; Weber, Funtan, et al., 2020, under review). They were assigned to the following treatment groups: Test formulation 1 (TF-PLACEBO) contained "Basiscreme DAC" (amphiphilic cream as published in the German Drug Codex; Table 1) with 20% medium-chained triglycerides; test formulation 2 (TF-BA) contained "Basiscreme DAC" with 20% medium-chained triglycerides and 1% BA; and test formulation 3 (TF-NVX207) contained "Basiscreme DAC" with 1% NVX-207. The test formulations were blinded by a number and letter code and unblinded after all analyses at the end of the study. The treatment was always performed by the same investigator (LAW). A crossover design was used to treat every horse with every formulation on the neck and undersurface of the tail for seven consecutive days, with a seven-day washout period between each formulation. The order of the formulations was randomized for each horse. Figure 1 gives an overview of the exact treatment sites. Treatment areas on the neck and control areas on the contralateral neck site were clipped 24 hr before each treatment period. The treatment sites were completely covered with about 1 g of the test formulations twice a day. If cream remnants from the previous treatment were still present, the skin was carefully cleaned with saline and swabs. The treatment and control sites in four horses (horses 3, 4, 7, and 8; randomly selected) were protected with a wound dressing ("Animal Soft," Snögg) and completely covered with "Fixomull stretch" (BSN medical GmbH). The covering on the neck was additionally attached with "AnimalPolster" (Snögg).

2.3 | Clinical examination and scoring

The horses were examined and scored by the first author (LAW), who was blinded to the treatment. The clinical examination and scoring were conducted twice a day during each treatment period and one day before and after each treatment period. The parameters obtained included behavior, posture, appetite, rectal temperature, mandibular lymph nodes, heart rate, mucous membranes, jugular vein filling, respiratory rate, auscultation of the thorax and the abdomen, and defecation. Summarized results from the clinical examination, skin areas treated and horses' behavior during test formulation application were scored in accordance with Table 2A, B, and C. Score results from the morning and evening examination were summed up daily in order to assess the burden for each horse. Horses with a score ≥11 on one day or ≥9 over three days, with a severely impaired general condition or severe skin reactions, were excluded from the study. The horses were clinically examined once a day on day 2–7 of each washout period but not scored.

TABLE 1 Ingredients of the "Basiscreme DAC" according to the German Drug Codex. Composition of 100 g cream

Purified aqua	40.0 g
Petrolatum	25.5 g
Propylene glycol	10.0 g
Medium-chained triglycerides	7.5 g
PEG-20-glyceryl stearate	7.0 g
Cetyl alcohol	6.0 g
Hydrogenated palm glycerides	4.0 g

2.4 | Sampling

Blood samples for complete blood counts and blood chemistry were taken in the morning of day 1 of each treatment period and in the morning of day 1 of each washout period. Blood chemistry included electrolytes (Na, K, Cl, Ca, Mg), bilirubin, glucose, urea, creatinine, bile acids, triglycerides, total protein, albumin, lactate, serum amyloid A and the enzymatic activity of the alkaline phosphatase, glutamate dehydrogenase, aspartate amino-transferase, γ-glutamyl transferase, creatine kinase, and lactate dehydrogenase. Furthermore, lithium-heparin plasma was analyzed for BA or NVX-207 content after the respective treatment, as described below.

Skin biopsies from the treatment and control sites were taken in the morning of day 1 of each washout period. The horses were sedated with butorphanol (0.01 mg/kg i.v.; "Butorgesic," cp-pharma, Burgdorf, Germany) and detomidine (0.01 mg/kg i.v.; "Cepesedan," cp-pharma). Mepivacaine ("Mepidor"; WDT) was used for local anesthesia. Three 8-mm punch biopsies were obtained from the neck (two from the treatment site, one control) and two 6-mm punch biopsies from the undersurface of the tail (one from the treatment site, one control) using single-use punch-biopsy instruments ("Dermal Biopsy Punch," WDT). Only one tail-control per horse was taken during the whole study to reduce the infection risk at this site. Biopsy wounds were cleaned, disinfected, and treated with ointment containing povidone-iodine ("Vet-Sept Salbe"; Albrecht GmbH) and aluminum spray ("Aluminiumspray"; aniMedica GmbH). Skin biopsies were fixed in 10% neutral-buffered formalin until further processing for histopathological examination. The second biopsy from the treated neck site was frozen at −20°C in aluminum foil until further processing for compound analysis.

2.5 | Quantification of BA and NVX-207 in the biopsy specimen and plasma

The skin sample processing was performed as described (Weber, Meißner, et al., 2020). Briefly, the frozen skin samples were cut

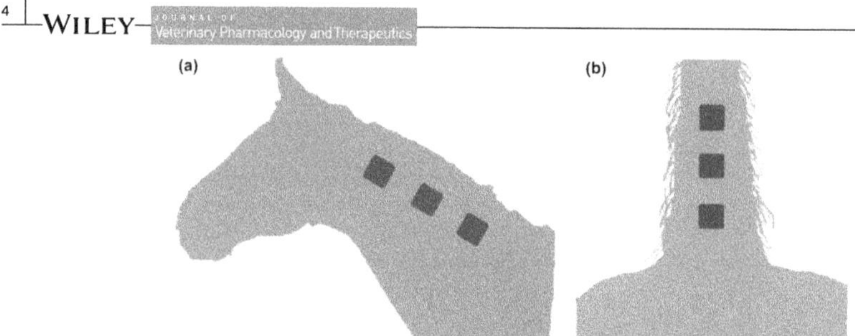

FIGURE 1 Schematic illustration of the treatment sites. (a) The three 5 × 5 cm treatment sites (one for each formulation) on the neck were located four, six and eight handbreadths caudal to C1 (atlas) and one handbreadth ventral to the crest. (b) The three 5 × 5 cm treatment areas on the ventral surface of the tail were located approximately one, two and three handbreadths caudal from the tail root. Note that the different treatment sites are not drawn to scale

TABLE 2 Scoring system

		Score
A	Clinical examination	0 = unremarkable 1 = mild alterations 2 = moderate alterations 3 = severe alterations
B	Skin reaction on treatment site	0 = skin is unremarkable 1 = skin is mildly reddened, warm, swollen, painful, mild desquamation 2 = skin is moderately reddened, warm, swollen, painful, moderate desquamation 3 = skin is severely reddened, warm, swollen, painful, severe desquamation
C	Behavior during test formulation application	0 = horse shows no defense movements or only mild muscle twitching 1 = horse is nervous; tail striking 2 = horse kicks, bites, tries to attempt application by active movement

Note: Horses were scored twice a day during treatment periods and one day before and after the treatments.

horizontally to the epidermis with a cryostat ("CryoStar™ NX70 Cryostat," Thermo Fisher) in skin slices (each with a thickness of 20 µm), after the first 10 µm (*stratum corneum*) had been separated due to possible cream residues. The skin slices were pooled at 5 × 20 µm, and the concentrations of BA and NVX-207 per 100 µm skin depth were consecutively analyzed by high-performance liquid chromatography (HPLC). The HPLC analysis for BA was performed as reported (Weber, Meißner, et al., 2020). Reverse phase analysis was conducted for NVX-207 determination using an Agilent 1100 system (Agilent) on a Luna® Omega column (3 µm, PS C18, 100 Å, 150 x 4.6 mm; Phenomenex) at 30 °C utilizing a gradient method with acetonitrile (0.1% HCOOH)(A):water (0.1% HCOOH)(B) at 1.1 ml/min (from 60% to 10% B within 7.50 min). The diode array detector was set at 200 nm.

Plasma samples were freeze-dried, extracted for 30 min with 1 ml methanol for NVX-207 samples and 1 ml ethanol for BA samples, and centrifuged with centrifugal filter units at 10T rpm for 10 min. A quantity of 40 µl of the supernatant was injected directly into the HPLC.

The detection limits of the HPLC methods were 0.1 µg/ml for both compounds (0.219 µmol/L for BA and 0.166 µmol/L for NVX-207).

2.6 | Histopathologic analysis of the biopsy specimen

The skin specimens fixed in neutral-buffered formalin were embedded in paraffin. Sections (each with a thickness of 3 µm) were stained with hematoxylin-eosin and evaluated histopathologically by a European specialist in veterinary pathology (CP) in a blinded process. Cell layers of the *stratum spinosum* were counted to assess the degree of epidermal hyperplasia. If there were up to twice as many cell layers compared to the corresponding control, the acanthosis was defined as "mild." If up to three times as many cell layers compared to the corresponding control were counted, the acanthosis was addressed as "moderate." More than three times as many cell layers compared to the control in the same location was defined as "severe acanthosis."

2.7 | Statistical analysis

Data analysis was performed using SAS 9.4m5 with the SAS Enterprise Guide, version 7.1 (SAS Institute Inc.). The quantitative parameters were checked for normal distribution by visual assessment of the Q-Q plots of the model residuals and calculating the Shapiro–Wilk test. Due to normal distribution of hematology and blood chemistry parameters, the effect of each treatment (TF-PLACEBO, TF-BA and TF-NVX207) for each blood parameter (difference between pre- and posttreatment) was calculated with a paired *t*-test for paired observations. A two-way analysis of variance with independent (covering) and correlated (treatments; all three treatments were performed on each horse with a time interval in between) measurements and the interaction between the two effects was calculated to compare the effects between treatment groups (TF-PLACEBO, TF-BA, and TF-NVX207) and covering (covering of treatment site vs. no covering of treatment site) on the influence of hematology and blood chemistry parameters (difference between pre- and posttreatment). The drug concentrations in the different skin depths were compared between BA and NVX-207, both with and without covering, using a two-way analysis of variance analogous to the evaluation of the blood parameters. The number of cell layers of the corresponding control was subtracted from the number of cell layers in the treated skin to compare the impact of the three different treatments (TF-PLACEBO, TF-BA, and TF-NVX207) and covering (covering of treatment site vs. no covering of treatment site) on the thickness of the *stratum spinosum*. In accordance with blood parameters, the differences were analyzed with a two-way analysis of variance. The Procedure Mixed was used for the linear model. The post hoc Tukey test was applied for multiple pairwise comparisons, while maintaining the experiential error rate. *p*-values $<.05$ were considered statistically significant.

3 | RESULTS

3.1 | Local and systemic tolerability of the topical treatments

Horse 8 had to be excluded from the study as it developed an acute lameness grade IV/V on the left front limb due to an orthopedic disorder (infected keratoma) on day 7 of the first washout period. The horse was treated with TF-NVX207 and, therefore, data for eight horses in the TF-NVX207 group and seven horses in the TF-PLACEBO and TF-BA group, respectively, were available.

All horses tolerated the repeated topical applications on both treatment sites very well (Score C: 0 for every horse in every treatment group). The mean score (±*SD*) for skin reactions after nine scoring days for each treatment was 3.4 (± 3.4) for TF-PLACEBO, 4.4 (± 3.9) for TF-BA and 1.4 (± 1.6) for TF-NVX207, with no difference observationally noted between horses with covered or uncovered treatment sites. The most common local side effects on the neck after all three treatments (TF-PLACEBO, TF-BA, and TF-NVX207) were mild erythema (TF-PLACEBO $n = 4$; TF-BA $n = 3$; TF-NVX207 $n = 1$), mild swelling (TF-PLACEBO $n = 3$; TF-BA $n = 1$; TF-NVX207 $n = 5$), and mild desquamation (TF-PLACEBO $n = 4$; TF-BA $n = 5$; TF-NVX207 $n = 3$). Palpation of the altered treatment site skin did not elicit a pain response. In most cases, side effects started during the fourth or fifth treatment day and resolved completely within the second to third day of the washout period. Mild alopecia on the neck ventral to the treatment site was observed in horse 1 (TF-BA) and horse 6 (TF-PLACEBO) at day 7 of treatment. The skin of the ventral tail was less affected compared to the cervical skin. Only horse 7 showed a mild erythema and desquamation on the skin of the tail from day four to seven when treated topically with TF-BA. No evidence of permanent cosmetic or functional deficits was observed in any horse on either treatment site (neck or tail).

Scores for the clinical examination revealed a good overall systemic tolerability of the topical treatment. The mean clinical score (±*SD*) for all horses after seven days of treatment with TF-PLACEBO was 0.6 (± 1.0), 0.4 (± 0.8) with TF-BA, and 0.3 (± 0.8) with TF-NVX207. Occasional observations of slightly increased heart or respiratory rates could always be linked to reasons other than the topical therapy. Horse 5 developed fever (max. 39.3°C) with a mild leukocytosis (max. 14.6 G/L; reference limits: 4.3–12 G/L) and increased serum amyloid A (max. 607 µg/ml; reference limit: <7 µg/ml) in the washout period after treatment with TF-NVX207. Biopsy wounds of this horse on the neck were mildly to moderately swollen and exudative. Wash samples from the guttural pouches for *Strep. equi* ssp. *equi* diagnostic and nasal swabs for Equine Influenza Virus type 1 and Equine Herpes Virus type 1 and 4 diagnostic were negative. The mare received metamizole (30 mg/kg i.v.; "Metamizol WDT"; WDT) twice and recovered within three days. The horse was suspended from the study for two weeks and then treated again to give her rest and ensure that the medication did not have any impact on the study results.

The blood results did not reveal any clinically relevant abnormalities, but there were occasional statistical differences. There was a statistically significant ($p < .01$) increase in lactate dehydrogenase after treatment with BA. While the lactate dehydrogenase of horse 4 changed from 351 to 311 U/L (reference range 0–235 U/L), the values of the other horses were within the reference range. Furthermore, a statistically significant decrease ($p < .05$) was observed in lymphocytes after treatment with BA. However, the blood values of the horses were within the reference range (20 – 45% of WBC), except for horse 1, which changed from 17.5% to 18.2%. A statistically significant increase ($p < .05$) was found in albumin and decrease ($p < .5$) in bile acids after treatment with NVX-207, but the blood values of all horses for both parameters were within the reference ranges (27–40 g/L for albumin and 0–12 µmol/L for bile acids). When the effects between treatment groups (TF-PLACEBO, TF-BA, and TF-NVX207) and covering (covering of treatment site vs. no covering of treatment site) on the influence of hematology and blood chemistry parameters were compared, a statistically significant difference was observed between the placebo and NVX-207 in hematocrit ($p < .05$) and erythrocytes ($p < .05$). However, the values of both parameters were within reference ranges (0.3–0.45 L/L for hematocrit and 5–10 T/L for erythrocytes).

3.2 | In vivo permeation profiles of BA and NVX-207 in equine skin and analysis of plasma samples

The skin biopsies differed in thickness, and each sample was processed at the cryostat as long as uniform sections were possible. Therefore, the skin depths analyzed ranged from 1,510 to 2,010 μm (median skin depth 2,010 μm). When the horse's skin was treated twice a day for seven consecutive days, NVX-207 and BA liberated from the carrier cream penetrated the *stratum corneum* and permeated through the epidermal and dermal skin layers. Noticeable, albeit not statistically significant ($p > .05$) differences in the amount of permeation and skin depth were found between the two compounds and a higher quantity of NVX-207 was detected up to a depth of 2,010 μm (Figure 2). Furthermore, higher concentrations of BA and NVX-207 were observed in the skin in horses with a covered treatment site compared to those with uncovered treatment sites, but differences were not statistically significant ($p > .05$) (Figure 2). The individual comparisons between NVX-207/covered treatment site and the other groups were significant (p-values <.05, .01 and .001) especially in the upper skin layers (up to 1,310 μm) with

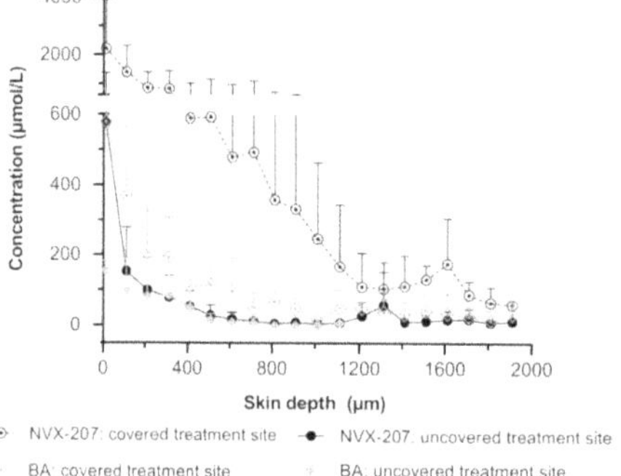

FIGURE 2 Concentration profiles of betulinic acid and NVX-207 in equine skin. Seven horses were treated topically on the neck with "Basiscreme DAC" +20% medium-chained triglycerides and 1% betulinic acid (BA) b.i.d. for seven consecutive days. Eight horses were treated with "Basiscreme DAC" and 1% NVX-207. The treatment site was covered in three (BA group) and four (NVX-207 group) horses. Data represent mean concentration (±*SD*) of BA and NVX-207 in cryostat skin slices at different skin depths determined by high-performance liquid chromatography. Each BA and NVX-207 concentration plotted corresponds to 100 μm skin depth, respectively. The active agent in the TF-BA group was found up to a median skin depth of 2,010 μm in horses with a covered treatment site (range from 1,310 to 2,010 μm) and up to a median skin depth of 760 μm in horses with an uncovered treatment site (range from 310 to 1,210 μm). The median permeated skin depth in horses treated with TF-NVX207 was 1,810 μm in both groups (covered and uncovered treatment site); however, it ranged from 1,510 to 2,010 μm in the covered and from 510 to 2,010 μm in the uncovered treatment site horses. No statistically significant difference between the groups could be shown

comparison-related error probability. Nevertheless, in the case of experiment-wise error rates (post hoc Tukey tests), the significances could not be shown due to the large number of tests, the small sample size, and the large scattering.

Neither BA nor NVX-207 were detected in any of the plasma samples.

3.3 | Histopathological examination of the skin

Histopathological changes were observed in the epidermis and dermis for all horses after all treatments (TF-PLACEBO, TF-BA, and TF-NVX207). The histopathological diagnoses were remarkably similar, regardless of whether the treatment site was covered or not. Most of the changes in the tail were very mild to mild, and those in the neck were mild to moderate. The *stratum corneum* on both treatment sites showed orthokeratosis in all horses after all treatments. Three horses additionally displayed multifocal parakeratotic areas of the neck (horse 7 after treatment with TF-PLACEBO, horse 6 after treatment with TF-BA, and horse 5 after treatment with TF-NVX20). A mild-to-moderate acanthosis of the *stratum spinosum* was observed in the cervical and tail skin after treatment with all three test formulations in all horses without any statistically significant difference ($p > 0.05$) between groups (TF-PLACEBO, TF-BA, and TF-NVX207/ covered treatment site vs. uncovered treatment site). The increase in the absolute number of *stratum spinosum* cell layers is shown in Table 3. Figure 3 illustrates the histopathological images of horse 2 after treatment with all three formulations as a representative example. One apoptotic keratinocyte each was found on the neck of horses 1 and 3 after treatment with TF-NVX207; the same was found on the neck of horses 1 and 2 after treatment with the placebo. A very slight to moderate, multifocal, perivascularly accentuated, lymphohistiocytic inflammation with a few neutrophils was observed in the superficial dermis of the neck and tail skin after all treatments (Figure 4).

4 | DISCUSSION

The aim of this placebo-controlled pilot study was to determine the concentration profiles of BA and NVX-207 in the skin of eight healthy horses when applied topically twice a day for seven consecutive days. The local and systemic tolerability of the compounds was also assessed. Higher concentrations of NVX-207 compared to BA were found in the skin. A good systemic tolerability and only mild local adverse effects were observed in all three groups (TF-PLACEBO, TF-BA, and TF-NVX207).

The transport of a therapeutic agent into the skin is a multi-step process, which has to be assessed carefully when developing a topical drug (Kalia & Guy, 2001; Luís et al., 2016). Firstly, the active compound needs to dissolve within and liberate from the pharmaceutical formulation. After penetrating and diffusing the skin's outermost layer and "major barrier"—the *stratum corneum*—mainly

 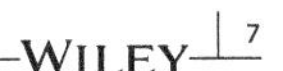

TABLE 3 Increase in *stratum spinosum* cell layers

	Cervical skin			Ventral tail skin		
	TF-PLACEBO	**TF-BA**	**TF-NVX207**	**TF-PLACEBO**	**TF-BA**	**TF-NVX207**
Uncovered treatment site	3 ± 1 (*n* = 4)	3 ± 1 (*n* = 4)	4 ± 1 (*n* = 4)	5 ± 3 (*n* = 4)	5 ± 2 (*n* = 4)	4 ± 2 (*n* = 4)
Covered treatment site	3 ± 2 (*n* = 3)	3 ± 1 (*n* = 3)	4 ± 2 (*n* = 4)	2 ± 4 (*n* = 3)	2 ± 2 (*n* = 3)	2 ± 1 (*n* = 4)

Note: Horses were treated topically on the neck and tail with a placebo (TF-PLACEBO), a 1% betulinic acid cream (TF-BA) or a 1% NVX-207 cream (TF-NVX207) b.i.d. for seven consecutive days in a crossover design. Cell layers in the *stratum spinosum* were counted. A mild-to-moderate acanthosis was observed in all horses after every treatment (TF-PLACEBO, TF-BA and TF-NVX207). Data represent the difference between cell layers of the treatment site and corresponding control (absolute numbers; mean ± *SD*), with positive values implying an increase in cell layers. There was no statistically significant difference ($p > .05$) between the groups (TF-PLACEBO, TF-BA and TF-NVX207/covered treatment site vs. uncovered treatment site).

via intercellular lipids, the therapeutic agent has to permeate the viable epidermis to reach the superficial dermis. The compound is absorbed in the dermis by local capillary blood vessels and an uptake into the systemic circulation takes place.

In the present study, BA and BA-derivative NVX-207 liberated from the carrier cream "Basiscreme DAC" with 20% medium-chain triglycerides (BA) or "Basiscreme DAC" only (NVX-207), penetrated the *stratum corneum*, and permeated the viable epidermal and dermal skin layers of equine cervical skin after topical application. Equine skin from the lateral thorax was used for in vitro permeation studies with BA and NVX-207 (Weber, Meißner, et al., 2020; Weber, Funtan, et al., 2020, under review). Regarding the in vivo study reported here, the horses were treated on the neck rather than the thorax to prevent the cream from being licked off by the animals. Concentration profiles were determined for the cervical skin only and, despite the 6-mm punch biopsy for histopathologic examination, no second biopsy was taken from the treated area underneath the tail. The rationale for this decision was the higher risk of infection at this location. The possible quantities of permeated active compounds calculated previously in skin slices of only 6 mm in diameter were below the detection limits of the HPLC methods (0.1 µg/ml). Thus, the risk of taking a second at least 8-mm large biopsy for substance quantification was considered inadequate. Equine neck skin is structurally similar to the skin of the thorax regarding epidermal and dermal thickness and the number of hair follicles (Scott & Miller, 2011; Wong, Buechner-Maxwell, & Manning, 2005) and, thus, good comparisons could be made with the in vitro results (Weber, Meißner, et al., 2020; Weber, Funtan, et al., 2020, under review). The concentration profiles of the substances in the tail skin can be expected to correspond, as there was no difference in the penetration of hydrocortisone, a substance with lipophilic properties close to BA and NVX-207, in clipped equine thoracic skin and nearly glabrous equine groin skin (Mills & Cross, 2006).

The area treated was covered with a patch in four horses in order to investigate whether this practice influences the permeation. The predilection sites for EMM are glabrous cutaneous regions, and the tumors are mainly found underneath the tail (Fleury et al., 2000; Seltenhammer et al., 2010). While not every part of the undersurface of the tail is in contact with the hind legs, the covering procedure may be necessary to prevent the cream from being rubbed off when treating a melanoma located laterally on the ventral tail. It was demonstrated that higher concentrations of the compounds were found in the covered compared to the uncovered skin, but differences were not statistically significant. Furthermore, permeated skin depths were deeper in horses with a covered treatment site. This may have been because the creams always remained at the desired location in these horses, even when they were rolling or laying in lateral recumbency for sleeping. Occlusion effects, which can occur due to covering of the skin or ingredients of the topical pharmaceutical formulation (e.g., propylene glycol, petrolatum), also could have had a positive influence on the permeation (Chang & Riviere, 1993; Prausnitz et al., 2012). Occlusion effects cause a hydration of the *stratum corneum* and, therefore, alter the barrier function of the skin (Chang & Riviere, 1993; Prausnitz et al., 2012).

After a treatment of seven days or 168 hr in vivo, the amount of BA and NVX-207 detected in the skin of horses with a covered treatment site was generally considerably higher than in the 24-hr in vitro samples (Weber, Meißner, et al., 2020; Weber, Funtan, et al., 2020, under review). On the one hand, this does not seem to be surprising due to the prolonged incubation time. On the other hand, it shows that although certain amounts of active agents are always transported away from the treatment site by capillary dermal absorption (Kalia & Guy, 2001), high concentrations of BA and NVX-207 can be achieved especially in the epidermis and superficial and partially deep dermis of equine skin in vivo. The concentration profiles of NVX-207 in horses with a covered and uncovered treatment site exceeded the respective concentration profiles of BA in vivo. By contrast, higher amounts of BA were found in isolated equine skin in vitro after an incubation of 24 hr in FDC experiments compared to the concentrations of NVX-207 (Weber, Meißner, et al., 2020; Weber, Funtan, et al., 2020, under review). This might be explained by a high affinity of both substances to the lipophilic *stratum corneum*, but there were differences in permeation rates through the viable, aqueous epidermis and dermis, which only became apparent in vivo after an application over a longer period of time (Guy & Hadgraft, 1984). The rapid penetration of the *stratum corneum* is followed by an accumulation of BA and NVX-207 in this skin layer, which leads to a reservoir effect—NVX-207 may permeate the hydrophilic epidermal and dermal tissue somewhat slower and is, therefore, absorbed more slowly by capillary blood vessels.

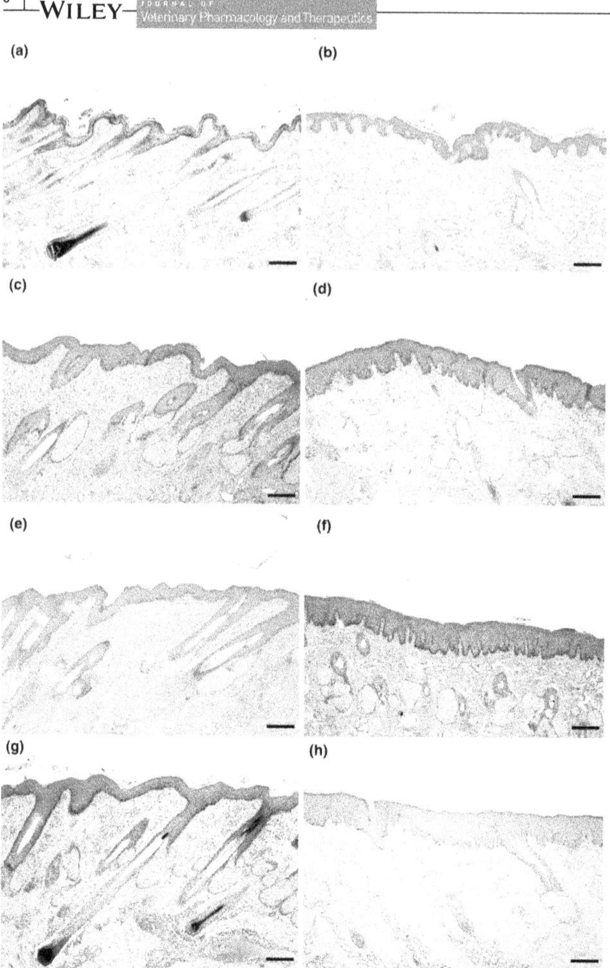

FIGURE 3 Hematoxylin and eosin staining of equine skin (horse 2). Histopathological images of cervical skin (left column—a, c, e, g) and ventral tail skin (right column—b, d, f, h) of horse 2 as a representative example of all eight horses enrolled in the study. The horse was treated topically twice daily for seven consecutive days with a placebo cream (c, d), a 1% betulinic acid cream (e, f) and a 1% NVX-207 cream (g, h). A different area of the neck or tail was treated for each test substance, and there was a one-week washout period between the individual test substances. Treatment sites were not covered on this horse. Pictures A and B show the untreated control sites. After the three treatment periods, a mild-to-moderate acanthosis of the *stratum spinosum* was observed in the neck and tail skin. A mild to moderate, multifocal, perivascularly accentuated, predominantly lymphohistiocytic inflammation was observed in the superficial dermis of both treatment sites (Hematoxylin and eosin, 40x, dimension bars correspond to a length of 200 μm)

Previously reported 96-h IC_{50} values with cytotoxic effects on EMM cells were reached in the deep dermis (up to 2,010 μm) for BA and NVX-207 in horses with a covered treatment site (Weber, Meißner, et al., 2020; Weber, Funtan, et al., 2020, under review). The amounts of BA and NVX-207 detected in horses with an uncovered treatment site exceeded the IC_{50} values for EMM up to a depth of 510 and 2,010 μm, respectively. While the skin sample thickness in previous FDC experiments was standardized and did not exceed 910 μm, the skin biopsy thickness in this study differed but never exceeded 2,010 μm. The active ingredients were found at the deepest skin depths analyzed, especially in horses treated with NVX-207 (covered and uncovered) and BA (covered). It is, therefore, possible that even deeper skin layers, which were not reached by the biopsy, had been permeated by the active ingredients. Taken together, the findings from the in vivo permeation study suggest that the treatment site should be covered in the topical application of BA and NVX-207. However, this must be confirmed by a larger sample size, as the differences between groups were not significant. Statistically, only a tendency was observed that a treatment with NVX-207 in combination with a covered treatment field increases the concentration in the skin compared to the other treatments. The covering could ensure that concentrations of the compounds, which have shown good effects against EMM cells at least in vitro, also reach lesions located in deeper equine skin layers. Nevertheless, a lack of correlation between the cell behavior in the natural microenvironment and under in vitro cell culture conditions is not uncommon, and

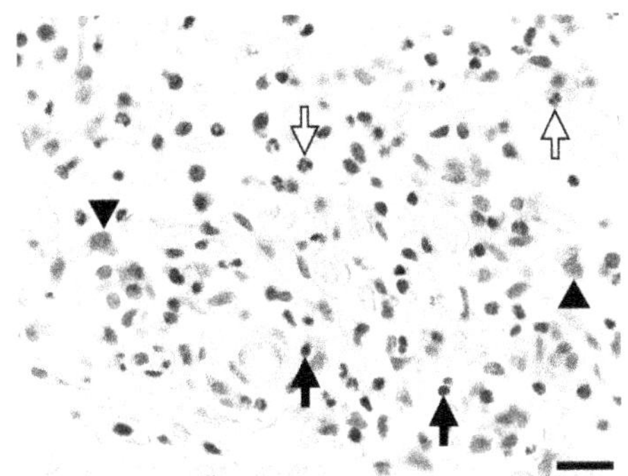

FIGURE 4 Hematoxylin and eosin staining of equine cervical skin after NVX-207 application (horse 2). The horse was treated topically twice daily for seven consecutive days on the neck with a cream containing 1% NVX-207. A moderate, multifocal, perivascularly accentuated, mainly lymphohistiocytic, partly neutrophilic inflammation was observed in the superficial dermis. Black arrows: Lymphocytes; black arrowheads: Macrophages; open arrows: Neutrophil granulocytes (Hematoxylin and eosin, 400×, dimension bar corresponds to a length of 20 μm)

cells in vivo may, therefore, be more robust against pharmacological influences (Hulsart-Billström et al., 2016; Wilson, Adelstein, Keegan, Barrett, & Kutz, 1996; Yao et al., 2014). Furthermore, EMM-induced changes in the skin structure (e.g., ulceration, encapsulation of the tumor) may alter the percutaneous permeation of the agents applied significantly compared to normal skin and, consequently, prospective clinical trials have to prove the antitumoral efficacy of the drugs.

Neither BA nor NVX-207 were detected in plasma samples by HPLC analysis at the end of each treatment period. Hematology and blood chemistry revealed no clinically relevant abnormalities. Consequently, it could be assumed that the risk of systemic adverse effects in horses after topical application is negligible due to the low systemic bioavailability of the compounds and an overall good systemic tolerability. It seems unlikely that the fever which developed in horse 5 in the washout period after NVX-207 application was related to the previous treatment, as the skin treated showed no clinical signs of inflammation. The biopsy wounds were mildly to moderately reactive one day after the biopsies were taken, which could possibly explain the disturbed general condition. No other infectious cause or ultrasonographic changes in the thorax or abdomen could be detected.

Mild erythema, mild swelling, and mild desquamation were the most common treatment-related local side effects clinically observed in the horses, regardless of whether the treatment site was covered or not. The local alterations were observed on the cervical skin and on the ventral tail skin only in one horse. These adverse effects became apparent not only after treatment with TF-BA and TF-NVX207 but also after treatment with the placebo. The skin alterations resolved within two to three days with no evidence of permanent cosmetic or functional deficits. Despite the clinical differences between the cervical and tail skin, interestingly, similar findings were obtained histopathologically for both treatment sites.

An epidermal hyperplasia or, more precisely, an acanthosis of the *stratum spinosum* and perivascularly accentuated lymphohistiocytic inflammation were the dominant findings in the histopathological examination of both the cervical and tail skin. The *stratum corneum* was not included in the data analysis. The cells of this skin layer are exposed to numerous exogenous influences and, therefore, the results may easily be falsified, for example, by the mechanical abrasion which can occur when a topical treatment is given twice a day. Epidermal hyperplasia is described as a common, nondiagnostic feature of virtually any chronic inflammatory process of the skin in horses (Scott & Miller, 2011). Another, albeit rather improbable, reason for the increased cell count of the *stratum spinosum* could be the so-called retention acanthosis, where the keratinocytes show a prolonged postmitotic lifespan and the epidermal turnover time is increased (Bullough, 1972; Lubach & Kietzmann, 1988). The perivascular dermatitis, as seen in nearly every horse after every treatment, could have arisen due to a hypersensitivity reaction to the creams applied (Scott & Miller, 2011). However, one would expect significantly more eosinophilic granulocytes and mast cells in real allergic or hyperergic processes than was the case with most of the biopsies in this study. It can be assumed that the clinical and histopathological skin alterations were associated with the ingredients of the "Basiscreme DAC" but not with the active compounds BA or NVX-207, as they were observed without a difference in all three treatment groups (TF-PLACEBO, TF-BA, and TF-NVX207). "Basiscreme DAC" is a pharmaceutical cream commonly used in humans and generally considered safe. However, it consists of, among others things, propylene glycol, cetyl alcohol, and glyceryl stearate, ingredients which have been demonstrated to induce mild skin irritations in animals such as mice and rabbits, partially even in lower doses than the ones in "Basiscreme DAC" (Johnson, 1988, 2004; Johnson et al., 2012). Furthermore, it has been demonstrated that an experimental acanthosis can be induced in guinea pigs after a seven-day treatment with yellow petrolatum (Born, 1969). Reports about safety assessments of pharmaceutical (or even cosmetic) ingredients in horses are rare and, therefore, no secure conclusion can be drawn from which ingredient(s) the local side effects originated in this study. Although evidence of a mild skin irritative potential was observed, a further use of the amphiphilic "Basiscreme DAC" as a vehicle for 1% BA and 1% NVX-207 should be considered, as a homogenous and stable distribution of the compounds in the cream is given (own laboratory controls; unpublished data). Furthermore, the previously mentioned findings from in vitro studies utilizing these creams (Weber, Funtan, et al., 2020, under review) were supported here by analytic in vivo experiments. Although the topical treatment with betulin, an alcohol related in structure to BA, was well tolerated in human patients suffering from actinic keratosis (Huyke, Laszczyk, Scheffler, Ernst, & Schempp, 2006; Huyke et al., 2008), further studies in humans are missing and, consequently, owners and veterinarians should wear gloves for safety reasons when treating the horses topically.

The relatively short treatment period and the small sample population in this pilot safety study limits the accurate tolerance predictability for a therapy over weeks and for a larger population and is, therefore, not comparable with an approval study. Nevertheless, good first insights into the concentration profiles and safety of BA and NVX-207 after topical application in horses were obtained.

5 | CONCLUSION

The results of this in vivo permeation and safety study indicate that high local concentrations of BA and NVX-207 can be reached in normal equine skin when applied topically twice a day for seven consecutive days. A covering of the treatment site seems to increase the drug concentration in the skin as well as the permeated skin depth, especially for NVX-207. Furthermore, it was demonstrated that the topical treatment of horses with both compounds is convenient and safe. Only mild local adverse effects were observed in all groups (TF-PLACEBO, TF-BA, and TF-NVX207), which suggests an association with ingredients in the carrier cream "Basiscreme DAC" but no causative effect of the compounds BA or NVX-207. This study supports the topical application of BA and NVX-207 in prospective clinical trials with horses suffering from EMM; however, the concentration profiles of the compounds may be altered in skin bearing tumors.

ACKNOWLEDGMENT

The project was funded by the Central Innovation Program of the German Federal Ministry for Economic Affairs and Energy. The authors would like to thank the animal care personnel of the Clinic for Horses, University of Veterinary Medicine Hannover, Foundation, for their support during the study. Open access funding enabled and organized by Projekt DEAL.

CONFLICT OF INTEREST

Manfred Kietzmann is a member of the editorial board of the Journal of Veterinary Pharmacology and Therapeutics.

AUTHORS' CONTRIBUTIONS

LAW contributed to the study design and data analysis, performed animal experiments and skin sample processing for HPLC analysis, and drafted and edited the manuscript. CP performed the histopathologic analysis of the skin biopsies. JK developed and performed the HPLC analysis. MK contributed to the study design and aided in data analysis and manuscript editing. KF contributed to the study design and aided in data analysis. KB prepared test formulations and aided in data analysis. KR performed the statistical analysis of the data. JMVC contributed to the study design, data analysis and aided in the manuscript editing. All authors read and approved the final manuscript.

ORCID

Lisa A. Weber https://orcid.org/0000-0001-6185-1595
Manfred Kietzmann https://orcid.org/0000-0001-5426-0631

REFERENCES

Baker, J. R., & Leyland, A. (1975). Histological survey of tumours of the horse, with particular reference to those of the skin. *Veterinary Record*, *96*(19), 419–422.

Born, W. (1969). Epidermal DNA synthesis in early experimental acanthosis of the guinea-pig. *Archiv Für Klinische Und Experimentelle Dermatologie*, *236*, 53–60. https://doi.org/10.1007/bf00504129

Bullough, W. S. (1972). The control of epidermal thickness. *British Journal of Dermatology*, *87*, 187–189. https://doi.org/10.1111/j.1365-2133.1972.tb00307.x

Chang, S. K., & Riviere, J. E. (1993). Effect of humidity and occlusion on the percutaneous absorption of parathion in vitro. *Pharmaceutical Research*, *10*(1), 152–155. https://doi.org/10.1023/A:1018901903243

Fleury, C., Bérard, F., Balme, B., & Thomas, L. (2000). The study of cutaneous melanomas in Camargue-type gray-skinned horses (1): Clinical-pathological characterization. *Pigment Cell Research*, *13*(1), 39–46. https://doi.org/10.1034/j.1600-0749.2000.130108.x

Fulda, S. (2008). Betulinic acid for cancer treatment and prevention. *International Journal of Molecular Sciences*, *9*(6), 1096–1107. https://doi.org/10.3390/ijms9061096

Galgon, T., Wohlrab, W., & Dräger, B. (2005). Betulinic acid induces apoptosis in skin cancer cells and differentiation in normal human keratinocytes. *Experimental Dermatology*, *14*(10), 736–743. https://doi.org/10.1111/j.1600-0625.2005.00352.x

Guy, R. H., & Hadgraft, J. (1984). Prediction of drug disposition kinetics. *Journal of Pharmaceutical Sciences*, *73*(7), 883–887.

Hulsart-Billström, G., Dawson, J. I., Hofmann, S., Müller, R., Stoddart, M. J., Alini, M., ... Oreffo, R. O. C. (2016). A surprisingly poor correlation between in vitro and in vivo testing of biomaterials for bone regeneration: Results of a multicentre analysis. *European Cells and Materials*, *31*, 312–322. https://doi.org/10.22203/eCM.v031a20

Huyke, C., Laszczyk, M., Scheffler, A., Ernst, R., & Schempp, C. M. (2006). Treatment of actinic keratoses with birch bark extract: A pilot study. *JDDG - Journal of the German Society of Dermatology*, *4*(2), 132–136. https://doi.org/10.1111/j.1610-0387.2006.05906.x

Huyke, C., Reuter, J., Rodig, M., Kersten, A., Laszczyk, M., Scheffler, A., ... Schempp, C. (2008). Treatment of actinic keratoses with a novel betulin-based oleogel. A prospective, randomized, comparative pilot study. *Journal Der Deutschen Dermatologischen Gesellschaft*, *7*(2), 128–133. https://doi.org/10.1111/j.1610-0387.2008.06865.x

Johnson, P. J. (1998). Dermatologic tumors (excluding sarcoids). *The Veterinary Clinics of North America: Equine Practice*, *14*(3), 625–658. https://doi.org/10.1016/S0749-0739(17)30190-6

Johnson, W. (1988). Final report on the safety assessment of cetearyl alcohol, cetyl alcohol, isostearyl alcohol, myristyl alcohol, and behenyl alcohol. *Journal of the American College of Toxicology*, *7*(3), 395–413. https://doi.org/10.1080/10915810802550835

Johnson, W. (2004). Final report of the amended safety assessment of glyceryl laurate, glyceryl laurate SE, glyceryl laurate/oleate, glyceryl adipate, glyceryl alginate, glyceryl arachidate, glyceryl arachidonate, glyceryl behenate, glyceryl caprate, glyceryl caprylate, glyc. *International Journal of Toxicology*, *23*(2), 55–94. https://doi.org/10.1080/10915810490499064

Johnson, W., Bergfeld, W. F., Belsito, D. V., Hill, R. A., Klaassen, C. D., Liebler, D., ... Andersen, F. A. (2012). Safety assessment of 1,2-glycols as used in cosmetics. *International Journal of Toxicology*, *31*, 147S–168S. https://doi.org/10.1177/1091581812460409

Kalia, Y. N., & Guy, R. H. (2001). Modeling transdermal drug release. *Advanced Drug Delivery Reviews*, *48*(2–3), 159–172. https://doi.org/10.1016/S0169-409X(01)00113-2

Liebscher, G., Vanchangiri, K., Mueller, T., Feige, K., Cavalleri, J. M. V., & Paschke, R. (2016). In vitro anticancer activity of Betulinic acid and derivatives thereof on equine melanoma cell lines from grey horses and invivo safety assessment of the compound NVX-207 in two horses. *Chemico-Biological Interactions, 246*, 20–29. https://doi.org/10.1016/j.cbi.2016.01.002

Lubach, D., & Kietzmann, M. (1988). Effects of treatment with dithranol, etretinate and a combination of dithranol and etretinate on epidermal metabolism and histology. Mouse tail assay. *Arzneimittel-Forschung/Drug Research, 38*(8), 1167–1170.

Luís, A., Ruela, M., Perissinato, A. G., Esselin, M., & Lino, D. S. (2016). Evaluation of skin absorption of drugs from topical and transdermal formulations. *Brazilian Journal of Pharmaceutical Sciences, 52*(3), 527–544. https://doi.org/10.1590/S1984-82502016000300018

Macgillivray, K. C., Sweeney, R. W., & Piero, D. (2002). Metastatic melanoma in Horses. *Journal of Veterinary Internal Medicine, 16*, 452–456.

MacKay, R. J. (2019). Treatment options for melanoma of gray Horses. *Veterinary Clinics of North America - Equine Practice, 35*(2), 311–325. https://doi.org/10.1016/j.cveq.2019.04.003

Mills, P. C., & Cross, S. E. (2006). Regional differences in the in vitro penetration of hydrocortisone through equine skin. *Journal of Veterinary Pharmacology and Therapeutics, 29*, 25–30. https://doi.org/10.1016/j.rvsc.2006.07.015

Moore, J. S. (2013). *A therapeutic practices established in human malignant melanoma in equine malignant melanoma [Doctoral dissertation]*. Virginia Polytechnic Institute and State University. Retrieved from https://pdfs.semanticscholar.org/a781/78ea35ccee0e98232936e88c863f891ee8a6.pdf

Moore, J. S., Shaw, C., Shaw, E., Buechner-Maxwell, V., Scarratt, W. K., Crisman, M., ... Robertson, J. (2013). Melanoma in horses: Current perspectives. *Equine Veterinary Education, 25*(3), 144–151. https://doi.org/10.1111/j.2042-3292.2011.00368.x

Nogueira, S. A. F., Torres, S. M. F., Malone, E. D., Diaz, S. F., Jessen, C., & Gilbert, S. (2006). Efficacy of imiquimod 5% cream in the treatment of equine sarcoids: A pilot study. *Veterinary Dermatology, 17*(4), 259–265. https://doi.org/10.1111/j.1365-3164.2006.00526.x

OECD (2004). *Guidance document for the conduct of skin absorption studies*. OECD Environmental Health and Safety Publications Series on Testing and Assessment No. 28. France. https://doi.org/10.1787/9789264078796-en

OECD/OCDE (2004). *Guideline for the testing of chemicals No. 428: Skin Absorption: in vitro Method (2004)*. France. https://doi.org/10.1787/20745788

Patterson-Kane, J. C., Sanchez, L. C., Uhl, E. W., & Edens, L. M. (2001). Disseminated metastatic intramedullary melanoma in an aged grey horse. *Journal of Comparative Pathology, 125*(2–3), 204–207. https://doi.org/10.1053/jcpa.2001.0481

Phillips, J. C., & Lembcke, L. M. (2013). Equine melanocytic tumors. *Veterinary Clinics of North America - Equine Practice, 29*(3), 673–687. https://doi.org/10.1016/j.cveq.2013.08.008

Prausnitz, M. R., Elias, P. M., Franz, T. J., Schmuth, M., Tsai, J.-C., Menon, G. K., ... Feingold, K. R. (2012). Skin barrier and transdermal drug delivery. *Medical Therapy, 5*(21), 2065–2073.

Reed, S., Bayly, W. M., & Sellon, D. (2018). *Equine internal medicine* (4th ed.). St. Louis, MO: Elsevier Inc.

Rodríguez, F., Forga, J., Herráez, P., Andrada, M., & Fernández, A. (1998). Metastatic melanoma causing spinal cord compression in a horse. *Veterinary Record, 142*(10), 248–249. https://doi.org/10.1136/vr.142.10.248

Scott, D. W., & Miller, W. H. (2011). *Equine dermatology* (2nd ed.). Maryland Heights, MO: Elsevier Saunders.

Seltenhammer, M. H., Simhofer, H., Scherzer, S., Zechner, P., Curik, I., Sölkner, J., ... Eisenmengr, E. (2010). Equine melanoma in a population of 296 grey Lipizzaner horses. *Equine Veterinary Journal, 35*(2), 153–157. https://doi.org/10.2746/042516403776114234

Selzer, E., Pimentel, E., Wacheck, V., Schlegel, W., Pehamberger, H., Jansen, B., & Kodym, R. (2000). Effects of betulinic acid alone and in combination with irradiation in human melanoma cells. *Journal of Investigative Dermatology, 114*(5), 935–940. https://doi.org/10.1046/j.1523-1747.2000.00972.x

Smith, S. H., Goldschmidt, M. H., & McManus, P. M. (2002). A comparative review of melanocytic neoplasms. *Veterinary Pathology, 39*(6), 651–678.

Soe, L., Wurz, G. T., Mäenpää, J. U., Hubbard, G. B., Cadman, T. B., Wiebe, V. J., ... DeGregorio, M. W. (1997). Tissue distribution of transdermal toremifene. *Cancer Chemotherapy and Pharmacology, 39*(6), 513–520. https://doi.org/10.1007/s002800050607

Sutton, R. H., & Coleman, G. T. (1997). Melanoma and the greying horse. *Rural Industries Research and Development Corporation, 97*(55), 1–27.

Traub-Dargatz, J. L., Salman, M. D., & Voss, J. L. (1991). Medical problems of adult horses, as ranked by equine practitioners. *Journal of the American Veterinary Medical Association, 198*(10), 1745–1747.

Valentine, B. A. (1995). Equine melanocytic tumors: A retrospective study of 53 Horses (1988 to 1991). *Journal of Veterinary Internal Medicine, 9*(5), 291–297. https://doi.org/10.1111/j.1939-1676.1995.tb01087.x

Valentine, B. (2006). Survey of equine cutaneous neoplasia in the Pacific Northwest. *Journal of Veterinary Diagnostic Investigation, 18*, 123–126.

VICH (2008). *Target animal safety for veterinary pharmaceutical products (VICH GL 43), European Medicines Agency – Veterinary Medicines and Inspections*. https://doi.org/10.1007/978-3-0346-0295-2_2

Weber, L. A., Funtan, A., Paschke, R., Delarocque, J., Kalbitz, J., Meißner, J., ... Cavalleri, J.-M.- V. (2020). In vitro assessment of triterpenoids NVX-207 and betulinyl-bis-sulfamate as a topical treatment for equine skin cancer. *PLOS ONE*. under review.

Weber, L. A., Meißner, J., Delarocque, J., Kalbitz, J., Feige, K., Kietzmann, M., ... Cavalleri, J.-M.- V. (2020). Betulinic acid shows anticancer activity against equine melanoma cells and permeates isolated equine skin in vitro. *BMC Veterinary Research, 16*(44), 1–9. https://doi.org/10.1186/s12917-020-2262-5

Willmann, M., Wacheck, V., Buckley, J., Nagy, K., Thalhammer, J., Paschke, R., ... Selzer, E. (2009). Characterization of NVX-207, a novel betulinic acid-derived anti-cancer compound. *European Journal of Clinical Investigation, 39*(5), 384–394. https://doi.org/10.1111/j.1365-2362.2009.02105.x

Wilson, D. A., Adelstein, E. H., Keegan, K. G., Barrett, B. A., & Kutz, R. R. (1996). In vitro and in vivo effects of activated macrophage supernatant on distal limb wounds of ponies. *American Journal of Veterinary Research, 57*(8), 1220–1224.

Wong, D., Buechner-Maxwell, V., & Manning, T. (2005). Equine skin: structure, immunologic function, and methods of diagnosing disease. *Compendium : Continuing Education for Veterinarians-North American Edition, 27*(6), 463–473.

Yao, M., Gu, C., Doyle, F. J., Zhu, H., Redmond, R. W., & Kochevar, I. E. (2014). Why is rose Bengal more phototoxic to fibroblasts in vitro than in vivo? *Photochemistry and Photobiology, 90*(2), 297–305. https://doi.org/10.1111/php.12215

Zalesińska, M. D., & Borska, S. (2019). Betulin and its derivatives – precursors of new drugs. *World Scientific News, 127*(3), 123–138.

How to cite this article: Weber LA, Puff C, Kalbitz J, et al. Concentration profiles and safety of topically applied betulinic acid and NVX-207 in eight healthy horses—A randomized, blinded, placebo-controlled, crossover pilot study. *J vet Pharmacol Therap*. 2020;00:1–11. https://doi.org/10.1111/jvp.12903

5. Manuscript IV:

Effects of topically applied betulinic acid and NVX-207 on early stage equine melanoma – A prospective, randomized, double-blind, placebo-controlled pilot study

Lisa A. Weber[1], Karsten Feige[1], Manfred Kietzmann[2], Jutta Kalbitz[3], Jessica Meißner[2*], Reinhard Paschke[4], Jessika-M.V. Cavalleri[5]

[1] Clinic for Horses, University of Veterinary Medicine Hannover, Foundation, Bünteweg 9, 30559 Hannover, Germany

[2] Department of Pharmacology, Toxicology and Pharmacy, University of Veterinary Medicine Hannover, Foundation, Bünteweg 17, 30559 Hannover, Germany

[3] Biosolutions Halle GmbH, Weinbergweg 22, 06120 Halle (Saale), Germany

[4] Biozentrum, Martin-Luther-University Halle-Wittenberg, Weinbergweg 22, 06120 Halle (Saale), Germany

[5] Equine Internal Medicine, University Equine Clinic, University of Veterinary Medicine Vienna, Veterinärplatz 1, 1210 Vienna, Austria

[*] Corresponding author

Under review at BMC Veterinary Research

Contribution to the manuscript:

LAW contributed to the study design, performed animal experiments and data analysis, and drafted and edited the manuscript. KF and MK contributed to the study design and data analysis. JK analyzed the active ingredient content in the formulations. JM and RP approved the manuscript critically for important intellectual content. JMVC contributed to the study design, data analysis and manuscript editing. All authors read and approved the final version of the manuscript.

Abstract

Background: The naturally occurring betulinic acid (BA) and its derivative NVX-207 induce apoptosis in equine melanoma cells *in vitro*. After topical (epicutaneous) application, high concentrations of the substances can be reached in healthy horse skin. Consequently, the topical therapy of the equine melanoma with BA or NVX-207 could be a feasible approach to treat early stages of the disease. The objective of the study was to gain insights into the effect and safety of topically applied BA and NVX-207 in horses with melanocytic tumors. The longitudinal, prospective, randomized, double-blind, placebo-controlled study protocol included eighteen Lipizzaner mares with early stage cutaneous melanoma assigned to three groups, each with six horses. One or two melanocytic lesions per horse were topically treated either with a placebo, 1 % BA or 1 % NVX-207 twice a day for 91 days. Caliper measurements, clinical examinations and blood tests were performed to assess the effects and safety of the treatment.

Results: The topical treatment was convenient and safe. After 91 days of treatment, 2 out of 8 tumors (25 %; 1 out of 6 horses) responded in the placebo group, 8 out of 12 tumors (67 %; 5 out of 6 horses) responded in the BA group and 4 out of 9 tumors (44 %; 3 out of 6 horses) responded in the NVX-207 group by means of tumor size and volume reduction.

Conclusions: The approach investigated might provide a feasible therapy to stabilize or even reduce tumor bulk in early stage equine melanoma cases. However, large-scale studies are required to verify these preliminary results.

Keywords: equine melanocytic tumor; horse; oncology; skin neoplasia; topical drug; triterpenoids

Introduction

The susceptibility to melanoma development in grey horses is high due to genetic mutations [1,2]. Early stages of the melanomas located mainly in the dermis frequently occur as single, black-pigmented, firm nodules in glabrous skin under the tail root, around the anus, perineum, external genitalia, in the lips and eyelids, or in rare circumstances at other locations [3–5]. Economic and functional problems such as interference with harness and breeding impairment have been reported [6,7] but more severe and life-threatening visceral signs can occur with disease progression and metastasis [8–13]. The often slow-growing nature of the tumors, the proximity to important anatomical structures such as nerves, vessels or the anal sphincter, and the currently challenging or inefficient therapeutic options have led many practitioners to advocate benign neglect of small melanocytic tumor masses in horses [8,9]. However, every equine melanocytic neoplasm should be considered potentially malignant and, therefore, worthy of treatment [8,9]. The topical (epicutaneous) treatment of equine melanomas could be a feasible approach to treat early stages of the disease. Topical therapies are characterized by their non-invasive nature and reduced systemic side effects [14,15]. Usually, they are affordable and can be performed with low logistical effort by the horse owners themselves, which reduces the stress factor on the horse significantly.

Betulinic acid (BA) is a pentacyclic lupane-type triterpenoid of plant origin [16]. Considerable amounts of the substance can be extracted from the bark of certain tree species, for example, the plane or the white-barked birch tree [16,17]. A wide range of pharmacological properties have been described for BA [18], among which the antitumoral features have been particularly studied [16,19,20]. The main antitumoral effects of the substance are based on the ability to trigger the mitochondrial pathway of apoptosis in cancer cells [21,22] to inhibit the eukaryotic topoisomerase I and II [23–25] and suppress the angiogenesis within the tumor [26–29]. Among a variety of BA derivatives, the compound NVX-207 has been identified as one of the most biologically active and pharmacologically significant agents [30–32]. The efficacy and mechanisms of BA and NVX-207 as potential therapeutics against equine melanoma were evaluated by *in vitro* cell culture experiments [32–34]. Reported findings suggest that BA and NVX-207 may achieve anticancer activity in equine melanoma cells due to cytotoxic and antiproliferative effects, whereby cell death is induced by apoptosis [32–34]. Concentration profiles of BA and NVX-207, both of which have been determined *in vitro* and *in vivo*, further indicated that the compounds' half-maximal inhibitory concentrations for equine melanoma cells can be achieved in healthy horse skin [33–35]. The *in vitro* and *in vivo* studies reported provide a promising basis for the use of BA and NVX-207 as topical drugs in clinical trials for equine melanoma treatment [32–35]. Consequently, the aim of this longitudinal, prospective, randomized, double-blind, placebo-controlled pilot study was to gain first insights into the effect and safety of BA and NVX-207 in horses with early stage melanoma after a 13-week long topical application.

Results

Tumor response

A total of 29 melanoma lesions (groups placebo n = 8; BA n = 12; NVX-207 n = 9) were treated twice a day for 13 weeks. The tumors were located on the ventral aspect of the tail or between the tail root and anus. The longest tumor diameter (length) measured on day 0 was 6.5 mm (median; min: 5.0 mm, max: 11.0 mm) in the placebo group. Tumors in the BA group had a median lenght of 5.5 mm (min: 3.0 mm, max: 12.0 mm). Tumor diameters in the NVX-207 group ranged from 4.0 to 9.0 mm with a median length of 6.0 mm.

A reduction in median absolute tumor volume was observed in every group. The median absolute tumor volumes in the placebo group reduced from 139.8 mm^3 (min: 62.5 mm^3, max: 550.0 mm^3) on day 0 to 117.0 mm^3 (min: 62.5 mm^3; max: 500.0 mm^3) on day 92. After treatment with BA, median tumor volumes decreased from 75 mm^3 (min: 32.0 mm^3, max: 864.0 mm^3) on day 0 to 51.3 mm^3 (min: 18.0 mm^3, max: 550.0 mm^3) on day 92. Median tumor volumes in the NVX-207 group decreased from 108.0 mm^3 (min: 32.0 mm^3, max: 288.0 mm^3) to 62.5 mm^3 (min: 32.0 mm^3, max: 288.0 mm^3). However, notably more tumors were categorized as "responded to treatment" in the BA and NVX-207 group than in the placebo group. After 91 days of treatment, 2 out of 8 tumors (25 %; 1/6 horses) responded to the treatment in the placebo group with a reduction of at least 1 mm in length and 1 mm in width compared to baseline measurements on day 0 (Figure 1). Eight out of 12 tumors (67 %; 5/6 horses) responded to the topical application of BA (Figure 2). In the NVX-207 group, 4 out of 9 tumors (44 %; 3/6 horses) decreased in length and width according to the definition of responsiveness (Figure 3). No new melanocytic lesions were detected in any of the horses during the treatment period.

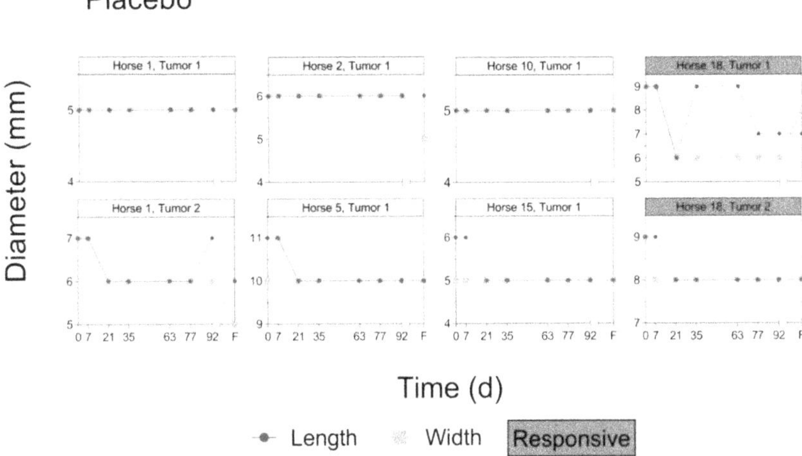

Figure 1 Tumor measurement values for the placebo group. Tumors were defined as "responsive to treatment" when there was a reduction of at least 1 mm in both dimensions (length and width) on day 92 compared to baseline measurements (day 0). F = values from follow-up measurements four months after the last treatment

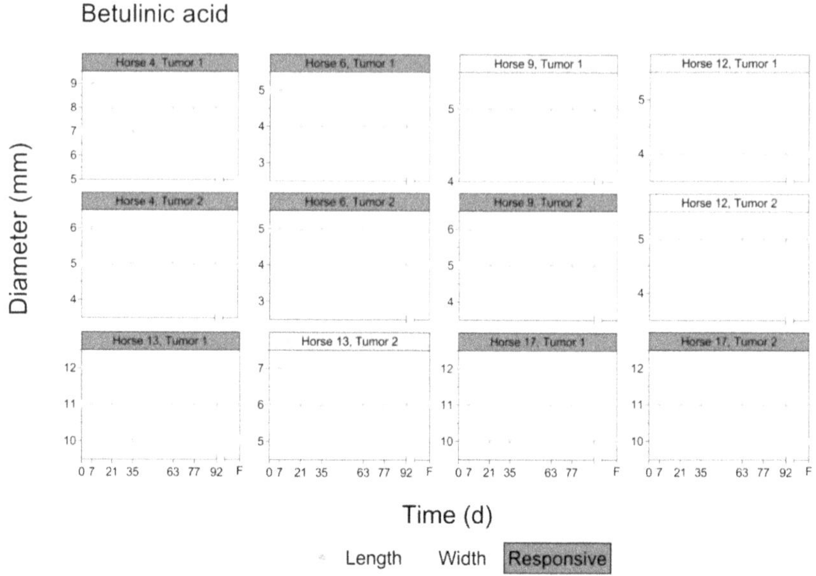

Figure 2 Tumor measurement values for the BA group. Tumors were defined as "responsive to treatment" when there was a reduction of at least 1 mm in both dimensions (length and width) on day 92 compared to baseline measurements (day 0). F = values from follow-up measurements four months after the last treatment

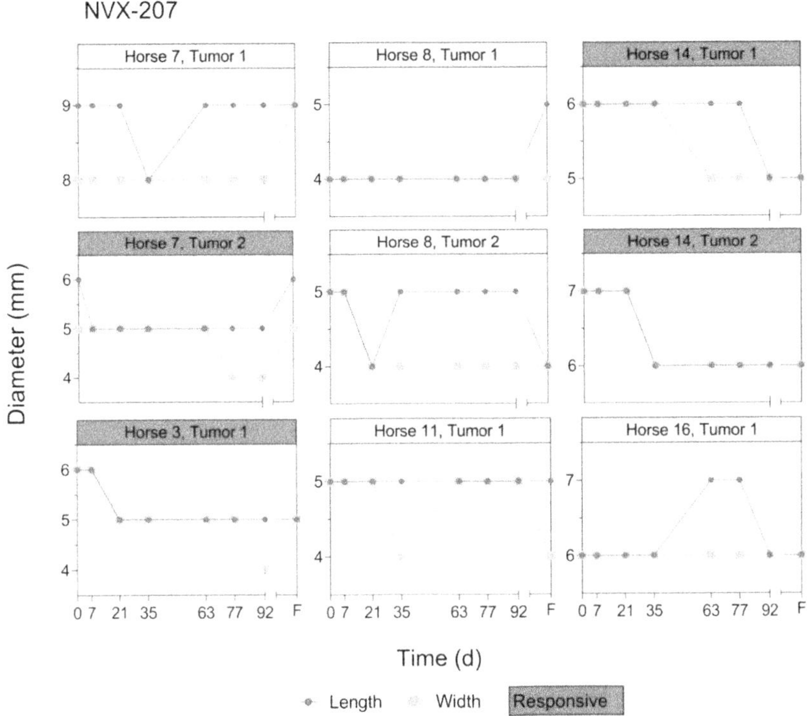

Figure 3 Tumor measurement values for the NVX-207 group. Tumors were defined as "responsive to treatment" when there was a reduction of at least 1 mm in both dimensions (length and width) on day 92 compared to baseline measurements (day 0). F = values from follow-up measurements four months after the last treatment

In the follow-up tumor measurements (Figures 1, 2, 3), tumor II of horse 7 (NVX-207 group) enlarged by 1 mm in both dimensions compared to values gained on day 92, whereas tumor I of horse 4 (BA group) and tumor II of horse 1 (placebo group) reduced by 1 mm in both dimensions. All other tumors were stable in size.

Clinical safety assessment of the treatment

All horses tolerated the topical drug application well and no active defense movements were observed during the treatments. The dressings covering the treatment areas reliably remained at the desired location. Based on the clinical examinations of the horses, the topical melanoma treatment was safe in all groups. Two horses developed a mild spasmodic colic on day 7 (horse

7; NVX-207 group) and on day 13 (horse 17; BA group). Both cases of colic were successfully treated with a single administration of mild spasmoanalgesics (50 mg/kg bodyweight metamizole sodium IV plus 0.2 mg/kg bodyweight butylscopolammonium bromide IV; "Novasul," Richter Pharma AG, Wels, Austria and "Buscopan compositum," Boehringer Ingelheim, Ingelheim, Germany). All pregnant mares gave birth to healthy foals. Blood results revealed no hematologic toxicity or clinically relevant abnormalities at any time point.

Depigmentation of the melanomas or the melanoma overlying skin was observed in 4 out of 8 tumors treated with the placebo (50 %; tumors of horses 1, 15, 18). The same was noted in 7 out of 12 tumors treated with BA (58 %; tumors of horses 4, 6, 13, 17) and 3 out of 9 tumors treated with NVX-207 (33 %; tumors of horses 7 and 14). An ulceration of melanoma II was observed in horse 6 from day 43 to day 70 after treatment with BA (Figure 4). The skin around the tumors treated was clinically unremarkable in all horses during the course of the study, except for horse 2 and 18 of the placebo group. In horse 2, the melanoma surrounding skin revealed isolated, depigmented areas from day 24 to day 86 of treatment. In horse 18, an isolated to extensive depigmentation of the skin around melanoma II was observed from day 16 to day 30 (Figure 5).

Four months after the end of the last treatment small, depigmented areas were apparent only in the two tumors of horse 17 (BA group). The skin of all the other horses was pigmented again.

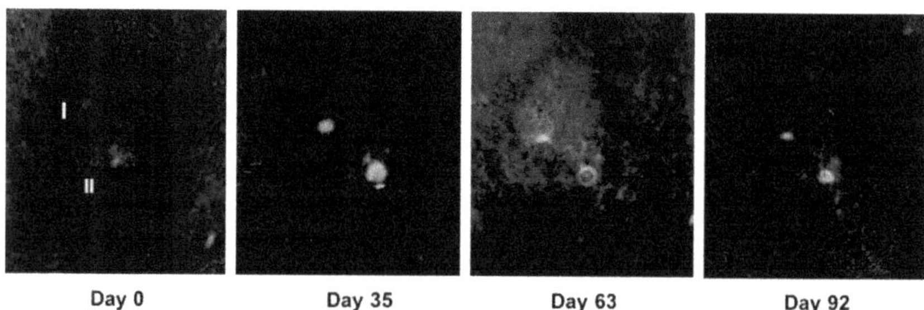

Figure 4 Clinical changes of melanoma I and II in horse 6 over time. The clinical changes of melanoma I and melanoma II (as indicated) on days 0, 35, 63 and 92 of the study. The tumors were treated twice a day with the 1 % BA preparation (in "Basiscreme DAC" + 20 % medium-chain triglycerides). In addition to the depigmentation of both tumors, an ulceration of melanoma II was occasionally observed from day 43 to day 70. Tumor volumes decreased from 63 mm^3 (melanoma I) and 63 mm^3 (melanoma II) on day 0 to 18 mm^3 (melanoma I) and 32 mm^3 (melanoma II) on day 92.

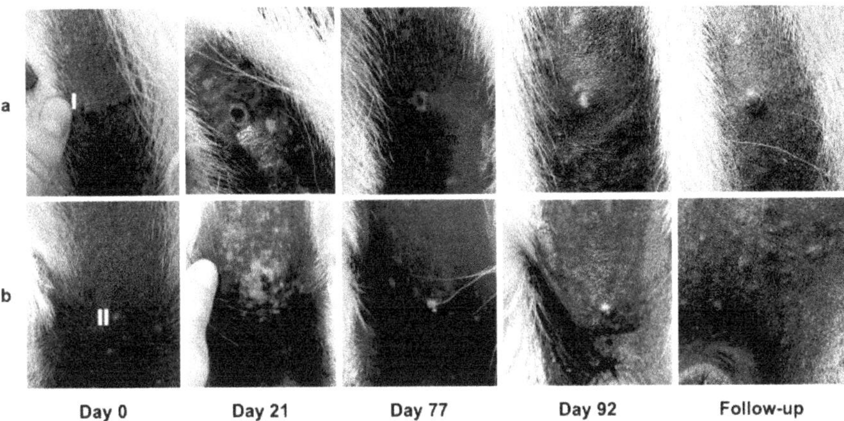

Figure 5 Clinical changes of melanoma I and II in horse 18 over time. The clinical changes of melanoma I (a) and melanoma II (b) on days 0, 21, 77 and 92 of the study and at follow-up examination. The tumors were treated twice a day with the placebo preparation ("Basiscreme DAC" + 20 % medium-chain triglycerides). A crust formed on melanoma I on the 13th day of treatment. When the crust was removed on day 19, the skin was ulcerated and the tissue underneath the crust was black and surrounded by an epithelial border. The tumor had decreased noticeably in size. The area was completely covered with partially depigmented skin on day 84. There was a reduction in the tumor volume by 239 mm^3 (melanoma I) and 109 mm^3 (melanoma II) at day 92 compared to the baseline volume. An isolated to extensive depigmentation of melanoma II and the surrounding skin was observed from day 16. Depigmentation was a temporary side effect.

Discussion

In the present pilot study, the topical application of 1 % BA or 1 % NVX-207 twice a day for 13 consecutive weeks in equine melanoma patients proved to be safe and was well tolerated. The topical therapy resulted in part in clinically visible and measurable changes in small melanoma lesions, which were reflected in skin depigmentation and reduction in tumor diameters and volumes. However, two tumors in the placebo group also showed a reduction in tumor size.

Although most melanocytic tumors in horses show a slow growth pattern for many years, more than two-thirds are thought to progress to malignancy [8,36]. Therefore, even small, early stage equine melanocytic tumors should be treated. Previously reported *in vitro* cell culture experiments and *in vitro* and *in vivo* permeation studies on unaltered horse skin indicated that the naturally occurring BA and its derivative NVX-207 may exert anticancer effects against equine melanoma [32–35]. The findings of this preceding work prompted further evaluation of safety and efficacy of the compounds in equine melanoma patients in the current study. Smaller tumors were deliberately treated to explore a potential therapy that can be used for early stages of the disease. Since changes of a few mm even in only one dimension (length or width) already have a large effect on the relative volume of small tumors compared to the relative volume of larger lesions, the relative volume changes were not indicated in the present study in order to prevent the results from being overinterpreted. It has been demonstrated previously that calculation of tumor volumes with caliper measurement and the formula used here correlates well with tumor volumes calculated using three-dimensional ultrasound measurements [37,38]. Eight out of 12 early stage cutaneous melanomas in 5 out of 6 horses responded to the topical therapy with BA in terms of a reduction in length and width of at least 1 mm. Although these first results after topical BA application on small equine melanocytic lesions are promising, the observations must be confirmed in larger studies with a more diverse horse population in order to be able to draw sound conclusions regarding the effectiveness of the substance in melanoma-affected horses. Modifications in the test formulation, such as increasing the concentration of the active ingredient or incorporating permeation enhancers that transport large amounts of the compound through the fibrous tumor capsule of equine melanomas to the tumor cells, could also have a positive effect on tumor volume regression.

Regarding the existing *in vitro* and *in vivo* data of NVX-207, it seems surprising that this derivative appears to have fewer anticancer effects on the tumors than its parent BA [30,32–35]. Its reported *in vitro* half maximal inhibitory concentrations which lead to antiproliferative and cytotoxic effects in equine melanoma cells are much lower than those determined for BA [32–34]. After 91 days of topical treatment with a cream containing 1 % NVX-207, 4 out of 9 melanocytic lesions in 3 out of 6 horses decreased in diameters and volume, but a complete tumor regression was not achieved. However, it should not be disregarded that tumor cells integrated in their native microenvironment can be much more robust against pharmacological influences than tumor cells cultivated under *in vitro* two-dimensional cell culture conditions and, therefore, a reliable transferability of *in vitro* to *in vivo* results is not always given [39,40]. In addition, permeation barriers, such as the firm tumor capsule often found around equine melanocytic tumors and which could hinder the active substance to diffuse into the tumor cell, are also missing [5,39,41]. While the half maximal inhibitory concentrations determined for equine melanoma cells were surpassed after topical application of 1 % NVX-207 in the epidermis, superficial and deep dermis of healthy horse skin [34,35], a less potent permeation into melanoma-affected skin could, therefore, further explain the only moderate effects of the compound in this study. It is also likely that tumors were located in the deep dermis and the NVX-207 applied topically may not have reached the full depth of the tumor invasion. An analysis of the NVX-207 content in the study medication a few weeks after the study termination revealed that the NVX-207 concentration had decreased only negligibly and a correlation between the reduced active ingredient content and reduced effectiveness can, thus, be excluded (own laboratory controls; data not shown).

The topical treatment of early stages of equine melanoma with 1 % BA and 1 % NVX-207 resulted in part in tumor volume and tumor diameter reductions and may represent an alternative to the frequently practiced approach of benign neglect of small solitary masses. Nevertheless, the results for lesions belonging to the BA und NVX-207 groups should be interpreted against the background that two tumors (both horse 18) in the placebo group also showed a decrease in tumor size that matched the definition of response to therapy. It was stated previously that no reports about spontaneous melanoma regressions in horses exist [37,42]. When the growth behavior of 59 untreated melanomas was investigated in 17 Lipizzaner stallions, the tumor volume increased by 0.14 % per day over an observation period of 162 days, but a slight reduction in tumor volume was sporadically observed in some lesions [43]. A trend in melanoma growth was observed in the placebo group of another study over only 64 days [44]. When the same pharmaceutical formulations as those used in this study were topically applied twice a day for seven consecutive days on eight healthy horses, an activation of the immune system by means of a perivascularly accentuated, lymphohistiocytic inflammation with a few neutrophils was observed in the superficial dermis of both the cervical and ventral tail skin [35]. As these alterations were noted in all treatment groups, an association with ingredients in the carrier cream "Basiscreme DAC" but no causative effect of the compounds BA or NVX-207 was suggested [35]. In the present study, the repeated topical application of the formulations for 13 consecutive weeks and the covering of the treatment areas could have led to an increased blood supply to the tumor area with increased immune cell infiltration. The presence of tumor-infiltrating lymphocytes has been associated with a favorable prognosis for human melanoma [45,46]. However, as no histopathological examinations of the melanomas treated with appropriate staining for vascularization markers or immune cell typing were performed in the present study, it remains unknown whether immunological adjuvant effects were involved in the tumor volume reduction. Since the tumor measurements were carried out by only one person, measurement variations can almost be excluded.

In equine sarcoids, treatment durations between three and 45 weeks are reported for the topical approach [47–50]. As there are currently no topical treatment options for the equine melanoma that rely on larger clinical evidence-based studies, the treatment regime in the current study could only be presumed. Previous determined *in vitro* data indicated that *in vivo* treatment regimens with short application intervals and long treatment durations could favorably influence the concentration and efficacy of BA and NVX-207 in the skin of equine melanoma patients [33,34]. In addition, the application interval of 13 weeks utilized in the recent study is similar to an 11-week topical application of frankincense oil to an Arabian mare with stage 3 equine melanoma, which resulted in a clear tumor volume reduction [51]. Whether an even longer application time of BA or NVX-207 leads to more notable clinical effects or even complete tumor regressions has to be investigated in further clinical studies. Interestingly, frankincense oil contains boswellic acids, pentacyclic triterpenoids comparable to BA and NVX-207, which were also shown to have *in vitro* and *in vivo* anticancer properties in human malignancies [51–55]. These data in conjunction with the results reported here could further indicate that prospective studies with this class of phytochemicals are auspicious in the field of equine skin cancer.

The topical melanoma treatment was safe and well tolerated in all groups as assessed by regular clinical examinations and serial blood sampling. The inconspicuous behavior may be related to the fact that the treatment did not cause painful skin inflammations. All horses showed an undisturbed general condition during the entire course of the study, apart from two horses with acute and medically resolved mild colic. Both horses that developed colic had a history of occasionally developing slight spasmodic colic at this time of the year. It seems very unlikely that the occurrence of colic was related to the topical melanoma treatment.

Depigmentation was occasionally observed in the skin surrounding and overlaying the tumors. The decreased amounts of melanin in the epidermis might be caused by toxic effects on the melanocytes or disturbed melanization due to the treatment [56]. Observations from follow-up examinations four months after the last treatment revealed that the depigmentation was a temporary side effect. While toxicity data of BA or NVX-207 for normal equine melanocytes are missing, a cytotoxicity of BA for human melanocytes by induction of apoptosis was described to varying degrees [57–59]. As the cases of depigmentation were also observed in the placebo group, an association with the ingredients of the amphiphilic carrier vehicle "Basiscreme DAC" is likely. With regard to the evidence of a mild skin irritative potential reported here and previously [35] and with respect to the fact that two tumors in the placebo group responded to the treatment, it is recommended to use another pharmaceutical formulation as a placebo and vehicle for BA and NVX-207 in future studies.

Although it is advantageous that topical medications are commonly affordable and can be easily applied by horse owners, the benefits of topical therapies appear to be limited to only the lesions treated and no systemic antitumor effects can be achieved. Melanomas of the lip seem unsuitable for a topical therapy because of the risk that the animal will lick off the cream or ointment and absorb it orally. By contrast, the treatment of melanomas located on the ventral tail and in the perianal region has been proven to be very feasible in this study. The study horses available for the present study had melanomas only at these regions. Future trials should evaluate the effect, safety and feasibility of the topical medication investigated when applied to melanomas located in different anatomical regions.

Particularly because there is no established gold standard treatment for equine melanoma, comparative study protocols should be considered for prospective studies. The phytochemical therapy introduced here and other described treatment modalities including surgery [60,61], radiation [62,63], (electro)chemotherapy [64–66] or immunotherapy [37,44,67,68] could be investigated. Moreover, approaches combining the aforementioned therapies with BA or NVX-207 as an adjunctive topical treatment could be the subject of further research.

Limitations of this pilot study include the usage of a single horse breed and sex, which limits predictability for a larger, more diverse population. In addition, due to the small number of animals, it was not further investigated whether the state of pregnancy in nine mares as well as the possibly different melanoma growth potential in horses with grey, flea-bitten or white coats could have an influence on the tumor response. Furthermore, no samples of the melanomas treated and surrounding skin were taken as this was not accepted by the stud management. Prospective studies should include tumor and skin biopsies in order to evaluate local treatment effects histophatologically and to measure compound concentrations in tumor tissues.

Conclusion

The results presented in this pilot study indicate that topical treatment of early stage equine melanoma with 1 % BA and 1 % NVX-207 twice a day over a period of 13 weeks is feasible and safe. A greater number of tumors responded to the therapy with BA and NVX-207 than tumors from the placebo group. This might suggest that this approach might be a potential therapy for early stage equine melanoma and, thus, reduce the health risks associated with the malignant degeneration of the tumors. However, these findings must be regarded as preliminary due to the limited group size and need to be replicated in a larger cohort. Modifications of the pharmaceutical formulations may further improve the clinical outcome.

Materials and Methods

Approval of the animal experiments

The longitudinal, prospective, randomized, double-blind, placebo-controlled study protocol was approved by the ethics committee of the University of Veterinary Medicine Vienna, Vienna, Austria and the Austrian Federal Ministry of Education, Science and Research in accordance with the Austrian Animal Welfare Law (BMBWF-Reference number: 68.205/0197-V/3b/2019). Informed consent was obtained from the stud management.

Horses

The study was performed between January and April 2020 at a stud farm in Austria. Eighteen white, flea-bitten or dappled Lipizzaner mares with cutaneous melanomas were included in this study (Table 1). The number of animals was determined by a power analysis using G*Power 3 [69].

Table 1 Characteristics and group assignment of the 18 Lipizzaner mares.

Horse ID	Treatment	Age (years)	Color	Melanoma stage*	Number of melanomas treated	Localization of the melanomas treated
1	Placebo	19	white	2	2	ventral tail
2	Placebo	14	white	2	1	ventral tail
5	Placebo	19	white	2	1	between tail root and anus
10	Placebo	9	dappled	2	1	between tail root and anus
15	Placebo	9	flea-bitten	2	1	ventral tail
18	Placebo	28	white	2	2	ventral tail
4	BA	17	white	2	2	ventral tail
6	BA	11	white	2	2	ventral tail
9	BA	12	flea-bitten	2	2	ventral tail
12	BA	18	white	2	2	ventral tail
13	BA	15	flea-bitten	2	2	ventral tail
17	BA	27	white	2	2	ventral tail
3	NVX-207	24	flea-bitten	2	2	ventral tail
7	NVX-207	20	grey	2	2	ventral tail

8	NVX-207	12	flea-bitten	2	2	ventral tail
11	NVX-207	14	grey	2	1	ventral tail
14	NVX-207	6	grey	2	2	ventral tail + between tail root and anus
16	NVX-207	9	grey	2	1	ventral tail

*Disease staging according to Moore et al. [9]

The median age of the horses was 14.5 years (range 6 to 28 years) and the median body condition score was 6 (range 4 to 8) according to the scoring scheme of Kienzle and Schramme [70]. Nine of the eighteen horses (horses 1, 5, 6, 9, 12, 13, 14, 15, 16) were in foal and the births of the foals were expected during or shortly after the study period. Horses were considered eligible for the study if they had not received a therapy for melanoma in the last three months and had cutaneous melanomas in localizations easy to treat (e.g. undersurface of the tail, udder in nonpregnant mares). Irrespective of the total number of melanomas identified on an individual horse, a maximum of two tumors per horse with a respective diameter of maximal 15 mm were treated. The tumors to be treated had to be easily distinguishable from each other and from other tumors. Clinical diagnosis was set at the beginning of the study on the basis of localization and gross appearance of the lesions in conjunction with the horses' signalment. Fine needle aspirations of tumor masses were performed in seven horses (horses 1, 5, 7, 12, 13, 17, 18) and clinical diagnosis was confirmed by cytological evaluation. For the other horses, the procedure would only have been possible under sedation, which was not permitted by the stud management. Medical histories were obtained before the instigation of the topical treatment and a thorough physical examination was performed on each horse to ensure eligibility for the trial. The animals were kept in groups of 15 to 25 horses in stables overnight and on a paddock during the day. After birth, mothers and foals were separated in individual boxes for about seven days before they were kept together in groups with other mares and foals in large stables. All horses were fed a mix of muesli, oats and mineral feed daily, the quantity of which depended on body weight and performance. They had *ad libitum* access to hay and water.

Topical treatment

The patients were randomized into three groups of six horses. Melanomas were topically treated with pharmaceutical test formulations (creams) which had been previously tested for tolerability on eight healthy horses and in which a homogenous and stable distribution of BA and NVX-207 had been shown [35]. Treatment was performed twice daily and consisted of topical application of either 1 % BA in "Basiscreme DAC" (amphiphilic cream as published in the German Drug Codex) with 20 % medium-chained triglycerides, 1 % NVX-207 in "Basiscreme DAC" or a placebo ("Basiscreme DAC" with 20 % medium-chained triglycerides) for 13 consecutive weeks (91 days). Each tumor was completely covered with the cream and protected with an appropriately sized wound dressing ("Animal Soft," Snögg, Vennesla, Norway), which was fixed with "Fixomull stretch" (BSN medical GmbH, Hamburg, Germany) to prevent the cream from being rubbed off (Figure 6).

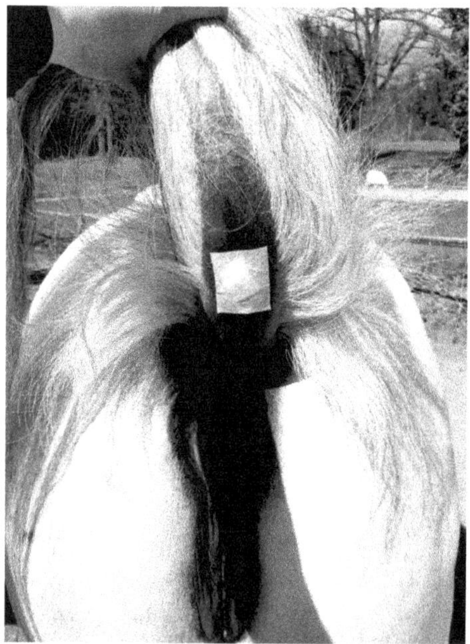

Figure 6 Covering the treatment site. Each tumor was treated topically with a placebo, a 1% betulinic acid cream or a 1% NVX-207 cream and protected with an appropriately sized wound dressing ("Animal Soft," Snögg, Vennesla, Norway), which was fixed with "Fixomull stretch" (BSN medical GmbH, Hamburg, Germany) to prevent the cream from being rubbed off.

Any cream residues from previous treatments were removed with a swab once a day. If necessary, the skin was degreased with swabs soaked in 70 % ethanol to ensure the fixation of the patches.

The study protocol stipulated that if the melanoma(s) disappeared completely before the end of the 13 weeks (tumor no longer palpable), the tumor was treated with the preparation assigned to it for another 14 days after tumor regression. The treatment was discontinued before the end of the 13 weeks if the tumor(s) grew aggressively.

The treatment was performed blinded by the first author (LAW). Horses 17 and 18 were treated by the stud's staff from day 56 to 83 of treatment due to restrictions in the context of the SARS-CoV-2 crisis. The identical-appearing study medication was packed in identically number-coded jars. The numerical code was unblinded after all analyses had been completed.

Clinical safety assessment of the treatment

Safety and tolerability of the topical treatment were evaluated by general clinical examinations, monitoring of the tumor and its surrounding clinically normal skin, and hematologic and blood biochemistry profiles. The animals were examined clinically prior to each topical application (twice a day) in the first week of treatment. Thereafter, a general clinical examination was performed twice at 14-day intervals (day 21 and 35) and then twice at 30-day intervals (day 63 and 92). The melanoma to be treated and the surrounding tissue were assessed daily for local inflammation, swelling, ulceration and depigmentation. Blood was collected on days 0, 7, 21, 35, 63 and 92 for a complete blood count and serum chemistry profile, including electrolytes (sodium, potassium, chloride, calcium, magnesium), urea, creatinine, total protein, albumin, lactate, serum amyloid A and enzymatic activity of the alkaline phosphatase, glutamate dehydrogenase, g-glutamyl transferase and creatine kinase.

The study protocol specified that treatment was discontinued if the horse showed moderate skin changes in the area treated for more than two days, if the horse showed mild abnormal physical examination parameters for five days or moderate abnormal physical examination parameters for three days, and in the case of significant illness or general deterioration in the condition of the horse.

Tumor response evaluation

Target lesions were photographed and the length (mm, longest diameter) and width (mm, perpendicular to length) were measured with calipers (CONNEX GmbH, Oldenburg, Germany) prior to treatment (day 0) and on days 7, 21, 35, 63, 77 and 92. Measurements were performed in duplicates. Tumor volume (mm^3) was calculated according to a formula described previously [37,38]: Tumor volume = length × width^2 × 0.5. Tumors were defined as "responsive to treatment" when there was a reduction of at least 1 mm in both dimensions (length and width) on day 92 compared to baseline measurements (day 0). All tumors were measured by the first author (LAW). Follow-up examinations of the horses and tumors were performed four months after the last treatment.

List of Abbreviations

BA = betulinic acid

Ethics approval and consent to participate

The study protocol was approved by the ethics committee within the University of Veterinary Medicine Vienna, Vienna, Austria, and the Austrian Federal Ministry of Education, Science and Research in accordance with the Austrian Animal Welfare Law (BMBWF-Reference number: 68.205/0197-V/3b/2019). Informed consent was obtained from the stud management. The study was carried out in compliance with the ARRIVE guidelines.

Consent for publication

Not applicable.

Availability of data and materials

The datasets analyzed during the current study are available from the corresponding author on reasonable request.

Competing interests

The authors declare that they have no competing interests.

Funding

The study was funded by the Central Innovation Program of the German Federal Ministry for Economic Affairs and Energy (Specific grant number: 16KN051526 BMWI). Further, this publication was supported by Deutsche Forschungsgemeinschaft and University of Veterinary Medicine Hannover, Foundation within the funding programme Open Access Publishing. The funders had no role in the design, analysis and reporting of the study.

Authors' contribution

LAW contributed to study design, performed animal experiments and data analysis and drafted and edited the manuscript. KF and MK contributed to study design and data analysis. JK analyzed the active ingredient content in the formulations. JM and RP approved the manuscript critically for important intellectual content. JMV contributed to study design, data analysis and manuscript editing. All authors read and approved the final version of the manuscript.

Acknowledgements

The authors kindly acknowledge the management and the horse grooms of the Spanish Riding School-Lipizzaner Stud Piber, in particular Mag. Alexandra Ferschel, for granting permission to conduct the study and great support during the study. The authors would also like to thank Dr. Konstanze Bosse (Skinomics GmbH Halle, Germany) for providing the test formulations.

The authors further thank Prof. Dr. Ilse Schwendenwein (Department for Pathobiology, University of Veterinary Medicine Vienna, Austria) for cytological evaluation of fine needle aspirations. The authors are grateful for valuable discussions with Dr. Barbara Pratscher (Division of Small Animal Internal Medicine, Department for Companion Animals and Horses, University of Veterinary Medicine Vienna, Austria) about the pathophysiology of equine melanoma.

References

[1] Sundström E, Imsland F, Mikko S, Wade C, Sigurdsson S, Pielberg G, et al. Copy number expansion of the STX17 duplication in melanoma tissue from Grey horses. BMC Genomics 2012;13:365. https://doi.org/10.1186/1471-2164-13-365.

[2] Rosengren Pielberg G, Golovko A, Sundström E, Curik I, Lennartsson J, Seltenhammer MH, et al. A cis-acting regulatory mutation causes premature hair graying and susceptibility to melanoma in the horse. Nat Genet 2008;40:1004–9. https://doi.org/10.1038/ng.185.

[3] Seltenhammer MH, Simhofer H, Scherzer S, Zechner P, Curik I, Sölkner J, et al. Equine melanoma in a population of 296 grey Lipizzaner horses. Equine Vet J 2003;35:153–7. https://doi.org/10.2746/042516403776114234.

[4] Fleury C, Bérard F, Balme B, Thomas L. The study of cutaneous melanomas in Camargue-type gray-skinned horses (1): Clinical-pathological characterization. Pigment Cell Res 2000;13:39–46. https://doi.org/10.1034/j.1600-0749.2000.130108.x.

[5] Seltenhammer MH, Heere-Ress E, Brandt S, Druml T, Jansen B, Pehamberger H, et al. Comparative histopathology of grey-horse-melanoma and human malignant melanoma. Pigment Cell Res 2004;17:674–81. https://doi.org/10.1111/j.1600-0749.2004.00192.x.

[6] Sutton RH, Coleman GT. Melanoma and the greying horse. RIRDC Res Pap Ser 1997;97:1–27.

[7] Johnson PJ. Dermatologic tumors (excluding sarcoids). Vet Clin North Am Equine Pract 1998;14:625–58. https://doi.org/10.1016/S0749-0739(17)30190-6.

[8] Macgillivray KC, Sweeney RW, Piero F Del. Metastatic Melanoma in Horses. J Vet Intern Med 2002;16:452–6.

[9] Moore JS, Shaw C, Shaw E, Buechner-Maxwell V, Scarratt WK, Crisman M, et al. Melanoma in horses: Current perspectives. Equine Vet Educ 2013;25:144–51. https://doi.org/10.1111/j.2042-3292.2011.00368.x.

[10] Patterson-Kane JC, Sanchez LC, Uhl EW, Edens LM. Disseminated metastatic intramedullary melanoma in an aged grey horse. J Comp Pathol 2001;125:204–7. https://doi.org/10.1053/jcpa.2001.0481.

[11] Smith SH, Goldschmidt MH, McManus PM. A Comparative Review of Melanocytic Neoplasms. Vet Pathol 2002;39:651–78.

[12] Rodríguez F, Forga J, Herráez P, Andrada M, Fernández A. Metastatic melanoma causing spinal cord compression in a horse. Vet Rec 1998;142:248–9. https://doi.org/10.1136/vr.142.10.248.

[13] Myrna K, Sheridan C. Melanocytic ocular and periocular tumours of the horse. Equine Vet Educ 2017:1–3. https://doi.org/10.1111/eve.12847.

[14] Luís A, Ruela M, Perissinato AG, Esselin M, Lino DS. Evaluation of skin absorption of drugs from topical and transdermal formulations. Brazilian J Pharm Sci 2016;52:527–44. https://doi.org/http://dx.doi.org/10.1590/S1984-82502016000300018.

[15] Prausnitz MR, Elias PM, Franz TJ, Schmuth M, Tsai J-C, Menon GK, et al. Skin Barrier and Transdermal Drug Delivery. Med Ther 2012;5:2065–73.

[16] Fulda S. Betulinic acid for cancer treatment and prevention. Int J Mol Sci 2008;9:1096–107. https://doi.org/10.3390/ijms9061096.

[17] Sarek J, Kvasnica M, Vlk M, Urban M, Dzubak P, Hajduch M. The Potential of Triterpenoids in the Treatment of Melanoma, Research on Melanoma - A Glimpse into Current Directions and Future

Trends. Rijeka, Croatia: InTech; 2011. https://doi.org/http://dx.doi.org/10.5772/57353.

[18] Ríos JL, Máñez S. New Pharmacological Opportunities for Betulinic Acid. Planta Med 2018;84:8–19. https://doi.org/10.1055/s-0043-123472.

[19] Pisha E, Chai H, Lee I-S, Chagwedera TE. Discovery of betulinic acid as a selective inhibitor of human melanoma that functions by induction of apoptosis. Nat Med 1995;1:1046–51. https://doi.org/10.1038/nm0495-365.

[20] Ali-Seyed M, Jantan I, Vijayaraghavan K, Bukhari SNA. Betulinic Acid: Recent Advances in Chemical Modifications, Effective Delivery, and Molecular Mechanisms of a Promising Anticancer Therapy. Chem Biol Drug Des 2016;87:517–36. https://doi.org/10.1111/cbdd.12682.

[21] Fulda S, Kroemer G. Targeting mitochondrial apoptosis by betulinic acid in human cancers. Drug Discov Today 2009;14:885–90. https://doi.org/10.1016/j.drudis.2009.05.015.

[22] Yang C, Li Y, Fu L, Jiang T, Meng F. Betulinic acid induces apoptosis and inhibits metastasis of human renal carcinoma cells in vitro and in vivo. J Cell Biochem 2018:8611–22. https://doi.org/10.1002/jcb.27116.

[23] Chowdhury RA, Mandal S, Mittra B, Sharma S, Mukhopadhyay S, Majumder HK. Betulinic acid, a potent inhibitor of eukaryotic topoisomerase I: identification of the inhibitory step, the major functional group responsible and development of more potent derivatives. Med Sci Monit 2002;8:254–60.

[24] Dillon LW, Pierce LCT, Lehman CE, Nikiforov YE, Wang YH. DNA topoisomerases participate in fragility of the oncogene RET. PLoS One 2013;8:1–15. https://doi.org/10.1371/journal.pone.0075741.

[25] Ganguly A, Das B, Roy A, Sen N, Dasgupta SB, Mukhopadhayay S, et al. Betulinic acid, a catalytic inhibitor of topoisomerase I, inhibits reactive oxygen species-mediated apoptotic topoisomerase I-DNA cleavable complex formation in prostate cancer cells but does not affect the process of cell death. Cancer Res 2007;67:11848–58. https://doi.org/10.1158/0008-5472.CAN-07-1615.

[26] Karna E, Szoka L, Palka JA. Betulinic acid inhibits the expression of hypoxia-inducible factor 1α and vascular endothelial growth factor in human endometrial adenocarcinoma cells. Mol Cell Biochem 2010;340:15–20. https://doi.org/10.1007/s11010-010-0395-8.

[27] Ren W, Qin L, Xu Y, Cheng N. Inhibition of betulinic acid to growth and angiogenesis of human colorectal cancer cell in nude mice. Chinese-German J Clin Oncol 2010;9:153–7. https://doi.org/10.1007/s10330-010-0002-1.

[28] Melzig MF, Bormann H. Betulinic acid inhibits aminopeptidase N activity. Planta Med 1998;64:655–7. https://doi.org/10.1055/s-2006-957542.

[29] Kwon HJ, Shim JS, Kim JH, Cho HY, Yum YN, Kim SH, et al. Betulinic acid inhibits growth factor-induced in vitro angiogenesis via the modulation of mitochondrial function in endothelial cells. Japanese J Cancer Res 2002;93:417–25. https://doi.org/10.1111/j.1349-7006.2002.tb01273.x.

[30] Willmann M, Wacheck V, Buckley J, Nagy K, Thalhammer J, Paschke R, et al. Characterization of NVX-207, a novel betulinic acid-derived anti-cancer compound. Eur J Clin Invest 2009;39:384–94. https://doi.org/10.1111/j.1365-2362.2009.02105.x.

[31] Csuk R. Betulinic acid and its derivatives: a patent review (2008 – 2013). Expert Opin Ther Pat 2014;24:913–23. https://doi.org/10.1517/13543776.2014.927441.

[32] Liebscher G, Vanchangiri K, Mueller T, Feige K, Cavalleri JMV, Paschke R. In vitro anticancer activity of Betulinic acid and derivatives thereof on equine melanoma cell lines from grey horses and invivo safety assessment of the compound NVX-207 in two horses. Chem Biol Interact 2016;246:20–9. https://doi.org/10.1016/j.cbi.2016.01.002.

[33] Weber LA, Meißner J, Delarocque J, Kalbitz J, Feige K, Kietzmann M, et al. Betulinic acid shows anticancer activity against equine melanoma cells and permeates isolated equine skin in vitro. BMC Vet Res 2020;16:1–9. https://doi.org/https://doi.org/10.1186/s12917-020-2262-5.

[34] Weber LA, Funtan A, Paschke R, Delarocque J, Kalbitz J, Meißner J, et al. In vitro assessment of triterpenoids NVX-207 and betulinyl-bis-sulfamate as a topical treatment for equine skin cancer. PLoS One 2020;15:1–22. https://doi.org/10.1371/journal.pone.0241448.

[35] Weber LA, Puff C, Kalbitz J, Kietzmann M, Feige K, Bosse K, et al. Concentration profiles and safety of topically applied betulinic acid and NVX-207 in eight healthy horses—A randomized, blinded, placebo-controlled, crossover pilot study. J Vet Pharmacol Ther 2020;00:1–11.

https://doi.org/10.1111/jvp.12903.

[36] Scott D. Neoplastic Diseases. In: Pedersen D, editor. Large Anim. Dermatology, Philadelphia, USA: W.B. Saunders Company; 1988, p. 448–52.

[37] Mählmann K, Feige K, Juhls C, Endmann A, Schuberth H-J, Oswald D, et al. Local and systemic effect of transfection-reagent formulated DNA vectors on equine melanoma. BMC Vet Res 2015;11:1–11. https://doi.org/10.1186/s12917-015-0422-9.

[38] Faustino-Rocha A, Oliveira PA, Pinho-Oliveira J, Teixeira-Guedes C, Soares-Maia R, Da Costa RG, et al. Estimation of rat mammary tumor volume using caliper and ultrasonography measurements. Lab Anim (NY) 2013;42:217–24. https://doi.org/10.1038/laban.254.

[39] Kapałczyńska M, Kolenda T, Przybyła W, Zajączkowska M, Teresiak A, Filas V, et al. 2D and 3D cell cultures – a comparison of different types of cancer cell cultures. Arch Med Sci 2016;14:910–9. https://doi.org/10.5114/aoms.2016.63743.

[40] Ferreira D, Adega F, Chaves R. The Importance of Cancer Cell Lines as in vitro Models in Cancer Methylome Analysis and Anticancer Drugs Testing. Oncogenomics Cancer Proteomics - Nov. Approaches Biomarkers Discov. Ther. Targets Cancer, vol. 3, InTech; 2013, p. 139–66. https://doi.org/10.5772/53110.

[41] Jain RK, Martin JD, Stylianopoulos T. The Role of Mechanical Forces in Tumor Growth and Therapy. Annu Rev Biomed Eng 2014;16:321–46. https://doi.org/10.1146/annurev-bioeng-071813-105259.

[42] MacKay RJ. Treatment Options for Melanoma of Gray Horses. Vet Clin North Am - Equine Pract 2019;35:311–25. https://doi.org/10.1016/j.cveq.2019.04.003.

[43] Peckary R. Average growth of melanomas in Lipizzaner horses and first test series for the development of an ELISA for detection of antibodies directed against human Tyrosinase in with human Tyrosinase vaccinated horses. University of Veterinary Medicine Vienna, 2019.

[44] Müller JMV, Feige K, Wunderlin P, Hödl A, Meli ML, Seltenhammer M, et al. Double-blind placebo-controlled study with interleukin-18 and interleukin-12-encoding plasmid DNA shows antitumor effect in metastatic melanoma in gray horses. J Immunother 2011;34:58–64. https://doi.org/10.1097/CJI.0b013e3181fe1997.

[45] Azimi F, Scolyer RA, Rumcheva P, Moncrieff M, Murali R, McCarthy SW, et al. Tumor-infiltrating lymphocyte grade is an independent predictor of sentinel lymph node status and survival in patients with cutaneous melanoma. J Clin Oncol 2012;30:2678–83. https://doi.org/10.1200/JCO.2011.37.8539.

[46] Fu Q, Chen N, Ge C, Li R, Li Z, Zeng B, et al. Prognostic value of tumor-infiltrating lymphocytes in melanoma: a systematic review and meta-analysis. Oncoimmunology 2019;8:1–14. https://doi.org/10.1080/2162402X.2019.1593806.

[47] Haspeslagh M, Jordana Garcia M, Vlaminck LEM, Martens AM. Topical use of 5% acyclovir cream for the treatment of occult and verrucous equine sarcoids: A double-blinded placebo-controlled study. BMC Vet Res 2017;13:1–6. https://doi.org/10.1186/s12917-017-1215-0.

[48] Stadler S, Kainzbauer C, Haralambus R, Brehm W, Hainisch E, Brandt S. Successful treatment of equine sarcoids by topical aciclovir application. Vet Rec 2011;168:1–4. https://doi.org/10.1136/vr.c5430.

[49] Nogueira SAF, Torres SMF, Malone ED, Diaz SF, Jessen C, Gilbert S. Efficacy of imiquimod 5% cream in the treatment of equine sarcoids: A pilot study. Vet Dermatol 2006;17:259–65. https://doi.org/10.1111/j.1365-3164.2006.00526.x.

[50] Pettersson CM, Broström H, Humblot P, Bergvall KE. Topical treatment of equine sarcoids with imiquimod 5% cream or Sanguinaria canadensis and zinc chloride – an open prospective study. Vet Dermatol 2020;31:471-e126. https://doi.org/10.1111/vde.12900.

[51] Moore JS. A Translational Study Evaluating the Uses of Diagnostic and Therapeutic Practices Established in Human Malignant Melanoma in Equine Malignant Melanoma [Doctoral dissertation]. Virginia Polytechnic Institute and State University, 2013.

[52] Kumar D, Kumar V, Jalwal P. Boswellic Acid- Potential tumors suppressant terpenoid -Photochemistry , Extraction and Isolation Methods -A comprehensive review study 2016;5:231–9.

[53] Frank MB, Yang Q, Osban J, Azzarello JT, Saban MR, Saban R, et al. Frankincense oil derived from Boswellia carteri induces tumor cell specific cytotoxicity. BMC Complement Altern Med 2009;9. https://doi.org/10.1186/1472-6882-9-6.

[54] Chen Y, Zhou C, Ge Z, Liu Y, Liu Y, Feng W, et al. Composition and potential anticancer activities of essential oils obtained from myrrh and frankincense. Oncol Lett 2013;6:1140–6. https://doi.org/10.3892/ol.2013.1520.

[55] Fung K, Suhail M, McClendon B, Woolley C, Young D, Lin H. Management of basal cell carcinoma of the skin using frankincense (Boswellia sacra) essential oil: A case report. OA Altern Med 2013;1:1–5. https://doi.org/10.13172/2052-7845-1-2-656.

[56] Scott DW, Miller WH. Equine Dermatology. 2nd ed. Maryland Heights: Penny Rudolph; 2011.

[57] Galgon T, Wohlrab W, Dräger B. Betulinic acid induces apoptosis in skin cancer cells and differentiation in normal human keratinocytes. Exp Dermatol 2005;14:736–43. https://doi.org/10.1111/j.1600-0625.2005.00352.x.

[58] Selzer E, Pimentel E, Wacheck V, Schlegel W, Pehamberger H, Jansen B, et al. Effects of betulinic acid alone and in combination with irradiation in human melanoma cells. J Invest Dermatol 2000;114:935–40. https://doi.org/10.1046/j.1523-1747.2000.00972.x.

[59] Surowiak P, Drag M, Materna V, Dietel M, Lage H. Betulinic acid exhibits stronger cytotoxic activity on the normal melanocyte NHEM-neo cell line than on drug-resistant and drug-sensitive MeWo melanoma cell lines. Mol Med Rep 2009;2:543–8. https://doi.org/10.3892/mmr_00000134.

[60] Rowe EL, Sullins KE. Excision as treatment of dermal melanomatosis in horses: 11 cases (1994-2000). J Am Vet Med Assoc 2004;225:94–6. https://doi.org/10.2460/javma.2004.225.94.

[61] Groom LM, Sullins KE. Surgical excision of large melanocytic tumours in grey horses: 38 cases (2001–2013). Equine Vet Educ 2018;30:438–43. https://doi.org/10.1111/eve.12767.

[62] Bradley WM, Schilpp D, Khatibzadeh SM. Electronic brachytherapy used for the successful treatment of three different types of equine tumours. Equine Vet Educ 2017;29:293–8. https://doi.org/10.1111/eve.12420.

[63] Henson FMD, Dobson JM. Use of radiation therapy in the treatment of equine neoplasia. Equine Vet Educ 2010;16:315–8. https://doi.org/10.1111/j.2042-3292.2004.tb00319.x.

[64] Théon AP, Wilson WD, Magdesian KG, Pusterla N, Snyder JR, Galuppo LD. Long-term outcome associated with intratumoral chemotherapy with cisplatin for cutaneous tumors in equidae: 573 cases (1995-2004). J Am Vet Med Assoc 2007;230:1506–13. https://doi.org/10.2460/javma.230.10.1506.

[65] Hewes C, Sullins KE. Use of cisplatin-containing biodegradable beads for treatment of cutaneous neoplasia in equidae: 59 cases (2000-2004). J Am Vet Med Assoc 2006;229:1617–22. https://doi.org/10.2460/javma.229.10.1617.

[66] Spugnini EP, D'Alterio GL, Dotsinsky I, Mudrov T, Dragonetti E, Murace R, et al. Electrochemotherapy for the Treatment of Multiple Melanomas in a Horse. J Equine Vet Sci 2011;31:430–3. https://doi.org/10.1016/j.jevs.2011.01.009.

[67] Phillips JC, Lembcke LM, Noltenius CE, Newman SJ, Blackford JT, Grosenbaugh DA, et al. Evaluation of tyrosinase expression in canine and equine melanocytic tumors. Am J Vet Res 2012;73:272–8. https://doi.org/10.2460/ajvr.73.2.272.

[68] Heinzerling LM, Feige K, Rieder S, Akens MK, Dummer R, Stranzinger G, et al. Tumor regression induced by intratumoral injection of DNA coding for human interleukin 12 into melanoma metastases in gray horses. J Mol Med 2000;78:692–702. https://doi.org/10.1007/s001090000165.

[69] Faul F, Erdfelder E, Lang A-G, Buchner A. G*Power 3: A flexible statistical power analysis program for the social, behavioral, and biomedical sciences. Behav Res Methods 2007;39:175–91. https://doi.org/10.3758/BF03193146.

[70] Kienzle E, Schramme SC. Body Condition Scoring and prediction of body weight in adult Warm blooded horses. Pferdeheilkunde 2004;20:517–24. https://doi.org/10.21836/PEM20040604.

6. General discussion

6.1. Summarized findings

With a growing awareness of animal welfare, an increasing population of horses being kept into older age and through better detection of tumors by horse owners and veterinarians there is considerable scientific and commercial interest in the discovery of new anticancer agents in equine medicine. Furthermore, cutaneous neoplasms are a significant cause of economic losses, morbidity and mortality in horses [6,7]. On this basis, the present thesis comprises four studies, all with the aim of contributing to the development of a topical therapy against equine skin cancer. The main focus of the investigations was the development of a novel drug for the treatment of EMM, however, the generated data can also contribute to further research projects dealing with treatment strategies for ES. Conducted cell culture experiments revealed antiproliferative, cytotoxic and apoptotic effects of BA, BA derivative NVX-207 as well as betulin derivative BBS against primary EMM and primary ES cells *in vitro*. Further *in vitro* and *in vivo* studies demonstrated a sufficient permeation of BA and NVX-207 into the epidermis and dermis of unaltered horse skin. A good systemic tolerability and only mild local, vehicle-related side effects were observed after topical application of BA and NVX-207 in eight healthy horses. Finally, the feasibility and effects of the topical BA and NVX-207 application in horses suffering from EMM were tested and these preliminary data indicated that this treatment approach – after further modifications of the pharmaceutical formulation – should be worth following up in a subsequent study with a larger number of patients included.

6.2. Interpretation of the findings

Currently, there is no topical medication for the treatment of EMM commercially available. For topical ES treatment, the results regarding the efficacy of topical acyclovir application are contradictory [69,86], imiquimod cream may temporarily cause severe local side effects [144] and for other topical therapies only anecdotal evidence exists [83,84]. Consequently, there is a need for a topical drug for the treatment of EMM and ES, backed by *in vitro* and in *vivo* evidence. The topical therapy of skin tumors in horses is a feasible approach, as neoplastic lesions at almost any localizations can be treated. Since the application is usually carried out by the horse owner in the environment to which the horse is accustomed, the treatment stress on the animal is significantly reduced. Besides, topical drug administration maximizes the local concentration of the agent and consequently increase the local efficacy [85]. Through the reduced systemic exposure of the drug, probable side effects to normal tissues are limited [87,145]. Furthermore, the non-invasiveness of the treatment and the good patient compliance has been extensively demonstrated in the present work.

Historically, natural products from botanical or animal sources have been used for virtually all medicinal preparations [9]. To this day, plant-derived substances or their synthetically modified analogues and derivatives are still a significant source for the development of new drugs and especially investigated within the area of cancer treatment [146,147]. The lupane-type triterpenes BA and betulin can be isolated from many plants, predominantly from the bark of birch and plane trees and have gained attention mainly due to their anticancer features [148,149]. On the basis of previously described cytotoxic and apoptotic effects on human and equine melanoma cells [96,109,113,150] and preliminary experiments within the framework of the current PhD project, the compounds BA, NVX-207 and BBS were used for the described investigations. The main focus of the *in vitro* and *in vivo* studies for the development of a topical drug against equine skin cancer was the clarification of penetration and permeation behavior of the compounds in equine skin as well as their safety and efficacy in the target species rather than the elucidation of detailed molecular pathways at the cellular level.

6.2.1. *In vitro cell culture experiments*

In a first step, *in vitro* experiments were carried out to determine whether the developed substances and the pharmaceutical test formulations had the potential to be used as topical medications for further *in vivo* experiments.

Cytotoxicity and proliferation assays. As described in manuscript I and II, the compounds BA, NVX-207 and BBS were demonstrated to exert significant antiproliferative and cytotoxic effects against primary EMM cells (MelDuWi and eRGO1), primary ES cells (sRGO1 and sRGO2) and primary equine dermal fibroblasts (PriFi1 and PriFi2) in a time- and dose-dependent manner. NVX-207 was by far the most potent drug that exerted the strongest effects on the different cells at each incubation time point in both CVS and MTS assay. While BA was more effective than BBS, the differences between these two compounds were not quite as marked. NVX-207 is synthesized by derivatization at C-3 (hydroxyl group) and C-28 (carboxylic group) positions of BA [137,151]. The present study demonstrated that simple modifications of the parent structure of BA can lead to a highly potent derivative. Thus, previous findings [96] on the cytotoxicity of BA and NVX-207 against EMM cells MelDuWi and MelJess after 96 h of incubation could be confirmed and widened by further methodical approaches (CVS and MTS assay), incubation times (5 h, 24 h, 48 h), cell types (sarcoid cells and fibroblasts) and a compound (BBS). Previously published cytotoxic activity on EMM cells was determined by the sulforhodamine B assay [96]. This might explain the differences of up to 10 µmol/L in the IC_{50} values for MelDuWi after 96 h of incubation with BA. While the sulforhodamine B dye binds to protein components of fixed cells independent of their active mitochondrial metabolic rate [152], the photometrical measurable formazan dye in the MTS assay is generated by mitochondrial dehydrogenases in metabolically active cells only [153]. Consequently, the MTS assay provides a more sensitive detection of reduced cell viability and, thus, lower IC_{50} values compared to those formerly reported were calculated in the present thesis (23.6 µmol/L vs. 33.1 µmol/L [96]). The IC_{50} values for MelDuWi after treatment with NVX-207 were proportionate (7.7 µmol/L reported here vs. 5.6 µmol/L [96]). In comparison to EMM cells eRGO1, higher concentrations of BA, NVX-207 and BBS were needed to exert antiproliferative and cytotoxic effects on MelDuWi, which therefore appear to be more robust against the active substances. This is a particular interesting observation since all the cells used for the cell culture experiments originated from different horses. Thereby, the results may indicate that EMM patients are not necessarily comparable and differences in the tumor response rates within a treatment group can be expected in future clinical studies with horses affected by this disease. This assumption has already been supported by the results of the *in vivo* efficacy study described in manuscript IV, in which 5/6 horses (67 % of tumors) in the BA group and 3/6 horses (44 % of tumors) in the NVX-207 group responded to the respective topical treatment. The ES cells sRGO2 were more sensitive to treatment with all three substances than sRGO1, but the differences were only marginal.

In vitro anticancer effects were observable in both EMM and ES cells as early as after 5 h of exposition to BA, NVX-207 or BBS. However, at this time point the quantity of cells affected by BA or BBS was mostly not high enough to calculate IC_{50} values with the applied software. The fact that 5-h IC_{50} values are available for NVX-207 in MTS and CVS assay for each type of cell investigated once again underlines the high *in vitro* efficacy of this substance. Generally, the data demonstrated that the antiproliferative and cytotoxic effects of the three substances investigated on equine skin tumor cells enhanced with an increased treatment duration in a dose-dependent manner. The lowest IC_{50} values were generated by CVS and MTS assay after 48 h of drug exposure for ES cells (no data available for 96 h) and 96 h for EMM cells. This information was particularly valuable for the study design of the reported *in vivo* efficacy trial, as it indicated that with a longer treatment period even lower concentrations of the active substances – as this was the case with the used 1 % creams – could be sufficient to trigger antitumor effects in equine skin cancer patients. Hence, these observations should also be incorporated into the design of future clinical studies with horses affected by EMM or ES.

Apoptosis assays. The study described in manuscript II is the first to investigate the induced form of cell death in ES and EMM cells after treatment with BBS and in ES cells after exposure to NVX-207. From the literature it is known that BA and NVX-207 induce apoptosis in various malignancies [96,115,125,137,149,154]. In previous investigations on EMM cells, BA and NVX-207 were demonstrated to activate both initiator caspases (caspase-8 and caspase-9) and the effector caspase-3 [96]. Furthermore, after treatment with BA and NVX-207 an accumulation of equine melanoma cells in the subG1-phase characterized by condensed chromatin and fragmented DNA and an externalization of phosphatidylserines to the extracellular side of the plasma membrane, also a characteristic feature of apoptosis, were reported [96]. Utilizing fluorescence-activated cell sorting (FACS), this controlled, highly regulated and therefore desired form of cell death could be confirmed for both types of equine skin cancer cells (EMM and ES) after treatment with NVX-207 and BBS. Within cell cycle analysis a clear increase of EMM and ES cells in the subG1-phase was detected after 48 h of drug exposure. Interestingly, BBS exerted greater apoptotic effects in ES cells as investigated by AnnexinV/propidium iodide staining compared to NVX-207, which was reverse in EMM cells. Together with the observation that sarcoid cells generally were more sensitive to BBS than melanoma cells in the sense that lower drug concentrations were needed to induce anticarcinogenic effects *in vitro*, this compound appears to be an interesting candidate for future studies dealing with treatment of ES. Even though apoptosis tests for sarcoid cells after treatment with BA were not explicitly carried out, such a mechanism of action can also be assumed for this compound. Still, this has to be confirmed in prospective cell culture investigations.

Effects on normal cells. Although various studies reported a selectivity of BA and NVX-207 to human cancer cells with no or only minimal toxic effects to human normal control cells including melanocytes [150], dermal fibroblasts [119,137], keratinocytes [137], peripheral blood lymphocytes [119,155], and umbilical vein endothelial cells [137], these findings could not be confirmed in the present studies. Both compounds were not revealed to exert a selective cytotoxicity or proliferation inhibition to EMM cells compared to normal equine dermal fibroblasts from healthy animals. Compared to ES cells, the unaltered cells were more robust to the compounds in CVS assay only. It is still remarkable that the proportion of necrotic cells, whether in altered or normal cell types, was below 2 % after a treatment of 48 h with NVX-207. In contrary to BA and NVX-207, the generated data gained on BBS indicated a selectivity of the compound to ES and EMM cells. In fact, EMM cells MelDuWi were the only exception from this observation in the MTS assay and revealed to be less affected by BBS than fibroblasts. Moreover, results from cell cycle analysis and AnnexinV staining revealed that BBS had mostly greater apoptotic impact in EMM and ES cells compared to fibroblasts. However, with regard to the broad array of pharmacological effects that are described for triterpenes and their derivatives [148], it seems not surprising, that non-cancerous equine skin cells could be affected by the compounds as well. Indeed, there are also some reports of BA's cytotoxicity in normal human melanocytes [154,156], low selectivity indices for dermal fibroblasts [120], and its induction of differentiation in keratinocytes, which is regarded as a specific form of apoptosis [154]. Studies concerning more detailed mechanisms of actions after treatment with triterpenes are rare in human unaltered cells and, to the best of the author's knowledge, have not yet existed for equine cells. As assessed by cell cycle investigations and AnnexinV/Propidium iodide staining in the present studies, NVX-207 and BBS induced apoptosis in equine dermal fibroblasts. Thus, with the FACS analysis reported here a valuable contribution could be made to this research topic. No apoptosis tests were performed on equine dermal fibroblasts after treatment with BA. Although similar results can be presumed, these must be confirmed in prospective cell culture experiments. BA has already found experimental application in rats [157] and mice [113,121,122,158]. NVX-207 was used in mice [137], dogs [137], and horses [96]. A good systemic tolerability for both compounds and only mild local adverse effects in dogs after NVX-207 therapy have previously been reported. Nevertheless, the results generated so far by the *in vitro* studies of the present work demonstrated that the tolerability of the substances after topical application on horse skin had to be investigated within the scope of the development of a topical drug against equine skin cancer. This was done in the studies described in manuscript III and IV and is discussed below.

Cell culture experiments – Conclusion and outlook. Taken together, the *in vitro* data gathered previously by Liebscher and colleagues [96] combined with our findings evaluating anticancer effects in EMM and ES cells supported further experiments with the three investigated compounds BA, NVX-207 and BBS. However, in order not to go beyond the scope of the project, it was decided that further studies would continue with the two more potent substances BA and NVX-207 only. Nevertheless, it should be emphasized at this point that the carbonic anhydrase IX inhibitor BBS is still a potential substance for the treatment of equine skin cancer, either alone or as an adjuvant therapeutic drug. The generated results proved it to be effective in both, EMM and ES cells, wherein the impact on ES cells was even more pronounced. Furthermore, of all, BBS was the compound that appeared to be the least toxic to healthy cells. In a study with human malignant melanoma cells a combination of proton pump- and carbonic anhydrase IX inhibitors did lead to enhanced anticancer effects in these cells *in vitro* [141]. Also, other carbonic anhydrase IX and XII inhibitors are discussed as versatile, emerging antitumor drugs [143]. Further studies are now necessary to confirm and expand these results in equine malignancies.

6.2.2. *In vitro permeation studies*

In a clinical setting, the topically applied BA and NVX-207 need to reach the tumor cells in the patient to be effective. Consequently, the next step was to find a way to transport the substances – dissolved in an appropriate vehicle – in sufficiently high concentrations into the horse skin.

Test formulations. The project partner Skinomics GmbH provided the 1 % pharmaceutical test formulations used for the *in vitro* permeation experiments on isolated equine skin and the *in vivo* safety and efficacy studies in horses. The amphiphilic "Basiscreme DAC" was selected as a carrier vehicle due to the fact that lipophilic substances like BA and NVX-207 can be easily incorporated and at the same time, as a standard vehicle in human medicine, it is considered to have little or no skin irritation potential. While a homogenous distribution of 1 % NVX-207 was given in "Basiscreme DAC" alone, 20 % medium-chained triglycerides had to be added to the BA formulation. The project partners performed long-term stability controls (including tests for chemical stability of the compounds, pH values, index of refraction, weight changes, gas evolution) and in-use controls, both at refrigerator temperature (4–8°C), room temperature (19–21°C) and 40°C with multiple batches of the creams. Both tests were performed up to three months. The unpublished results from the various tests demonstrated that a homogenous and stable distribution of the compounds in the test formulations was given at refrigerator and room temperatures.

Penetration and permeation in isolated equine skin. With the FDC cell experiments and subsequent compound detection in the skin samples via HPLC analysis it was demonstrated that both BA and NVX-207 were able to penetrate the *stratum corneum*, the major barrier for transdermal drugs, and permeate through the epidermal and dermal strata of unaltered equine thoracic skin. The concentrations reached after 30 minutes and 24 h of incubation exceeded the 24-h IC_{50} values for ES and EMM cells even in the deepest skin layers examined (up to 810 µm). Due to differences in skin structure in a range of animal species [159–162], it was of great advantage that the skin of the target species could be used for *in vitro* FDC studies. Nevertheless, the results should be interpreted against the background of some limitations. Melanomas in grey horses are mainly localized in the dermis or subcutis of nearly glabrous cutaneous regions [17,19,20]. In the light of the *in vitro* results generated in this thesis, it appears that after topical application of BA or NVX-207 melanomas located in the superficial and partially deep dermis would come into contact with sufficiently high amounts of the compounds and, therefore, might be affected by their cytotoxic and antiproliferative effects. However, the concentration profiles of the drugs may be altered in skin affected by tumors – either because the permeation of the drugs through the tumor tissue itself is altered or because skin changes caused by tumor growth could influence it. On the one hand, tumor ulcerations could have a positive influence on the permeation rates, as the *stratum corneum* has no longer to be overcome. This phenomenon was already suspected in an ulcerated EMM that responded well to topical frankincense oil therapy [55]. On the other hand, fibrous tumor capsules, which envelop some EMM [20], may protect the tumor tissue from being permeated by the compounds. Epidermal alterations like hyperplasia and hyperkeratosis as well as rete peg formation is frequently observed in verrucous and mixed sarcoids, but often not present in occult and nodular lesions [65]. The epidermal thickening could negatively influence the concentration profiles of the topically applied drugs [90] and the penetration and permeation of the active agents in the latter two forms of ES could, therefore, rather be comparable with the data gained from unaltered horse skin. Hence, one major limitation of the present work is the lack of data about the concentration profiles of the compounds in EMM or ES affected skin. Due to technical reasons, the utilization of a standardized protocol with tumor skin was not possible during the present thesis project. However, it is highly recommended to solve this task in future projects. As in previously reported FDC experiments with isolated equine skin [93,161,163], the integument from the lateral thorax was used in the present work. In view of the fact that ES often occur in the saddle area and saddle girth position [56], the choice of the lateral thorax skin for the FCD protocol does not need to be justified for this type of tumor. On the contrary, a minor limitation of the utilized FDC protocol is the use of equine thoracic skin rather than the skin of EMM predilection sites (ventral tail, perianal region, external genitalia, etc.). Nonetheless, the concentration profiles of hydrocortisone, a substance with lipophilic properties similar to BA and NVX-207, did not differ significantly in clipped equine thoracic skin and nearly glabrous groin skin [163]. In addition, as groin skin and EMM predilection site skin are equivalent in morphology [2,164] the permeated amounts of the compounds hence can be expected to be comparable.

In vitro permeation studies – Conclusion. Summarized, the gained *in vitro* data in equine skin cancer cells and the *in vitro* concentration profiles in isolated equine skin as described in manuscript I and II indicated BA and NVX-207 as promising candidates for the topical treatment of equine skin cancer and substantiated further study of BA and NVX-207 in horses. Although *in vitro* FDC studies can be predictive for *in vivo* penetration and permeation data [87,94], they cannot provide information about the amount of a compound that is eliminated from the skin by capillary dermal blood vessels, as isolated skin lacks of circulation. Besides, the whole complexity of a biological system, including the metabolism, distribution and elimination of a drug, cannot be reproduced by FDC experiments [87,94]. Therefore, it was of great advantage that the concentration profiles and safety of the active substances could subsequently be determined *in vivo* in the target species, as described in manuscript III.

6.2.3. *In vivo safety and permeation studies*

As the calculated IC_{50} values for ES and EMM cells were reached in isolated equine skin after topical application of the respective 1 % test formulations, for animal welfare reasons and with regard to possible cytotoxic effects on normal skin cells, the utilization of test formulations with higher concentrations was not justifiable. Consequently, further *in vivo* studies were carried out with the previously investigated creams.

Study horse compliance. All eight horses enrolled in the *in vivo* safety and permeation study (manuscript III) tolerated the topical treatment on the neck and ventral tail twice a day very well and no defense movements during drug application were noted at any time. Two of the mares were previously used as brood mares and were therefore used to having their tails lifted by humans. The other six horses represented a mixed population, demonstrating that repeated topical treatments of the ventral tail should also be associated with good patient compliance in other horses.

Concentration profiles. After seven days of treatment with the test formulation containing either 1 % BA or 1 % NVX-207, the permeated amounts of the compounds in the cervical horse skin *in vivo* exceeded the concentrations found in isolated equine skin after 24 h of incubation noticeably. Moreover, in horses with a covered treatment site the concentrations of BA and NVX-207 surpassed the 96-h IC_{50} values for equine skin cancer cells even in the deep dermal skin layers (up to 2010 μm). While this was also true for NVX-207 in horses without covered treatment sites, the required concentrations for BA in horses with uncovered treatment sites were only reached in the superficial dermis. According to these findings, two important statements regarding the concentration profiles of BA and NVX-207 in equine skin could be generated by the *in vivo* permeation study. First, even though certain amounts of topically applied drugs are always transported away from the treatment site by capillary dermal absorption [91], high concentrations of BA and NVX-207 can be achieved especially in the epidermis and superficial and partially deep dermis of equine skin *in vivo*. Second, the results indicated that the treatment field should be covered after topical application of the 1% test formulations. Although this hypothesis could not be statistically confirmed, the results suggested that by covering the treatment area both, the amount of the active ingredient in the skin increased and deeper skin layers could be reached by the compounds. On the one hand, this could be explained by the fact that the cream remained more reliably at the treated location, regardless of whether the horses were rolling or laying in lateral recumbency. Nevertheless, it was frequently observed that there were still cream residues on the skin between the applications even in horses with uncovered treatment areas. Therefore, on the other hand, occlusion effects caused by covering of the skin or ingredients in the cream (e.g. propylene glycol, petrolatum) could be the reason for the increased permeation [90,165]. Swelling of the keratinocytes leads to a distention of the intercellular spaces, and polar and nonpolar substances can penetrate through "pores" in the *stratum corneum* interstices more rapidly [90].

Local and systemic safety. One major issue in cell culture research with BA and NVX-207 concerned the compounds' cytotoxicity to normal equine dermal fibroblasts. Within the scope of the current study, the local and systemic safety of the substances was therefore also investigated clinically as well as by blood tests and histopathological examinations.

Theoretically, regarding the reported IC_{50} values for equine dermal fibroblasts, the achieved BA and NVX-207 concentrations in the skin were high enough to have cytotoxic and antiproliferative effects on these skin cells. However, although these influences on equine dermal fibroblasts were described *in vitro* and apoptosis- and necrosis-like effects and increased differentiation in human keratinocytes and melanocytes were observed after *in vitro* treatment with BA [150,154,156], only a very few apoptotic keratinocytes and no necrotic cells were detected histopathologically in the skin samples after treatment with NVX-207 and the placebo formulation. These findings are in line with other studies demonstrating that fibroblasts grown under three-dimensional cell culture conditions are less sensitive to toxic agents than those grown in monolayers [166,167]. In contrast to their cultivation as monolayers on a plastic cell culture flask, the equine dermal fibroblasts in intact skin are surrounded by extracellular matrix and interact with the matrix macromolecules [168]. The matrix molecules, mainly structural proteins and proteoglycans, strongly influence cell physiology and affect cell responses to stimuli, whereby they improve the ability of fibroblasts to withstand stresses [166–168].

The topical treatment of horse skin with 1 % BA in "Basiscreme DAC" and 20 % medium-chained triglycerides and 1 % NVX-207 in "Basiscreme DAC" as well as the placebo preparation ("Basiscreme DAC" and 20 % medium-chained triglycerides) was occasionally (n= 1 – 5 / 8 horses; depending on test formulation) associated with local adverse reactions like mild erythema, mild swelling and mild desquamation at the cervical skin. The tail skin showed mild alterations in one horse only. These skin alterations resolved within two to three days with no evidence of permanent cosmetic or functional deficits in any affected horse. An acanthosis of the *stratum spinosum* and perivascularly accentuated lymphohistiocytic inflammation were the dominant findings in the histopathological examination of both the cervical and tail skin. As these clinical and histopathological reactions were observed without a difference in all three treatment groups (BA, NVX-207 and placebo), an association with the ingredients of the carrier cream "Basiscreme DAC" but not with the active compounds BA or NVX-207 could be assumed. No secure conclusion could be drawn from which ingredient(s) the local side effects originated in this study due to the fact that reports about safety assessments of pharmaceutical or even cosmetic ingredients in horses are rare. However, the ingredients propylene glycol, cetyl alcohol and glyceryl stearate contained in "Basiscreme DAC" have been demonstrated to induce mild skin irritations in animals such as mice and rabbits, partially even in lower doses than the ones found in the test formulations [169–171].

The unremarkable systemic clinical examinations of the horses, no abnormalities in hematology and blood chemistry as well as the fact that neither BA nor NVX-207 was detected in any of the plasma samples at the end of each treatment period, attest a low systemic bioavailability and an overall good systemic tolerability of the substances after topical application in horses.

The repeated intralesional injection of NVX-207 was well tolerated in two horses suffering from EMM [96]. This study in conjunction with the results reported in this thesis indicate that the topical application of BA and NVX-207 should be considered as safe in equine patients. Although a mild skin irritative potential was observed, a further use of the amphiphilic "Basiscreme DAC" as a vehicle for 1 % BA and 1 % NVX-207 was decided. The previous findings from the *in vitro* permeation experiments have been supported by the *in vivo* study. Furthermore, the long-term studies on the stability and homogeneous distribution of the active ingredients in the cream were positive.

Safety and permeation studies – Limitations and conclusion. Limitations of the *in vivo* safety and permeation studies included the short treatment period and small sample population. This is presumably the reason why only a statistically tendency could be shown that covering of the treatment site seems to increase the drug concentration in the skin as well as the permeated skin depth, especially for NVX-207. Moreover, the data do not allow any conclusion to be drawn about the safety of the therapy over several weeks and for a larger population. Nonetheless, valuable first insights into the concentration profiles and safety of topically applied BA and NVX-207 in horses were obtained.

Despite these promising preliminary *in vivo* results, it should be considered that the permeation behavior of the substances in skin affected by EMM or ES can be changed for reasons already explained above. In addition, tumor cells integrated in their *in vivo* native microenvironment can be more robust against pharmacological influences than those cultivated under two-dimensional *in vitro* cell culture conditions [172–174]. Therefore, still no reliable statement about the efficacy of topically applied BA and NVX-207 on equine skin cancer patients could be made with the data generated so far (manuscript I, II and III).

6.2.4. *In vivo efficacy study*

To assess the *in vivo* antitumoral effects of the topically applied drugs, the investigated test formulations were used in eighteen horses suffering from early stage EMM (manuscript IV). A further clinical trial with ES patients was not possible within the present PhD project, but the investigations described in manuscript I, II and III provide a good basis to advance the development of a topical therapy for this form of equine skin cancer. The various clinical and histopathological manifestations of ES might explain the differences that are encountered in the treatment responses to the multiple described therapy options [65,84]. Accordingly, there is still a great need for research on risk factors, etiology, pathogenesis and possible treatment approaches to the disease in order to develop reliable and evidence-based therapies. So far, no studies have been published about the mechanisms of action of BA, NVX-207 or BBS in ES cells. The data from this work may thus help to develop a way in which the tumors could be controlled on the cellular level with topically applied phytochemicals – either as a monotherapy or as part of a combinational treatment protocol. Treatment durations between three weeks and eight months are reported for the topical approach in ES [69,83,86,144]. An appropriate treatment period for sarcoids treated with the formulations investigated here must be determined in future studies with ES patients.

As shown by the study described in manuscript IV, the topical application of 1 % BA or 1 % NVX-207 twice a day for 13 consecutive weeks (91 days) in EMM patients proved to be convenient and safe. The topical therapy resulted in part in clinically visible und measurable changes in early stage EMM lesions, which were reflected in skin depigmentation and reduction in tumor volumes. Eight out of 12 tumors responded to treatment in the BA group and four out of nine tumors reduced in volume in the NX-207 group. However, two tumors in the placebo-group showed also a reduction in tumor size. The treatment regime for the efficacy study could only be presumed, as there are currently no topical treatment options for EMM patients that rely on larger clinical evidence-based studies. Chemotherapy usually works best in fast growing tumors with high mitotic indices [11]. Due to the often slow growth rate of early stage EMM, it could, therefore, be speculated that a long-lasting treatment duration had to be applied [7,21,30]. Results from *in vitro* cell culture experiments indicated that the longer the cancer cells are in contact with the compounds, the less concentration of BA and NVX-207 is required to exert antiproliferative and cytotoxic effects. In addition, another study reported an 11-week long topical treatment of frankincense oil to a large EMM lesion, which led to a noticeably volume reduction of the tumor [55].

Tumor selection. Early stage melanomas were selected for the efficacy study described here. In accordance with the clinical EMM classification system published by Moore and colleagues [21], the disease of all horses treated within the study were classified as EMM stage 2 (multiple, slow growing tumors < 2 cm without metastasis). However, it should be noted that no metastasis control was performed in the study horses. A reliable metastasis control in the living horse is currently not possible due to limited diagnostic possibilities. Prospective EMM classification systems should be modified accordingly. Generally, it is advisable to consider early therapy of all accessible small EMM and ES lesions. Late stages of EMM have an increased risk of malignancy [7,21] and, besides, the therapy of larger EMM and ES tumors is known to be challenging or even impossible [21,84]. Hence, for the current study it was inferred that smaller tumors are (at least theoretically) more susceptible to the topical phytochemotherapy because there are fewer and more easily accessible tumor cells to kill [11]. Consequently, the rationale for the decision to treat small EMM lesions was the consideration that the deepest cells within the tumor mass core in large tumors might be physically protected from the effects of the topically applied BA and NVX-207. Probably the drugs would have been resorbed from outer tumor cell layers and no sufficient levels would have reached the deepest cells. To address this hypothesis, prospective FDC experiments with melanoma-affected skin have to be carried out. Concentration profiles of the compounds within tumors of different sizes could be determined, once the methodology for these kinds of experiments is established and standardized protocols are available.

Efficacy in EMM patients. Even though treated EMM lesions were small, only tumor size reductions but no complete tumor remissions could be achieved after treatment with BA or NVX-207. It is likely that tumors were located in the deep dermis and the topically applied drugs may have not reached the full depth of the tumor invasion – even though the treatment fields were continuously covered, which does, as shown in study III, increase the amount of drug in the skin and permeated skin depth. Furthermore, tumor induced skin changes like the fibrous tumor capsule, which was palpable around many lesions, could have negatively influenced the permeation of the drugs. Besides – as already mentioned above – chemotherapies work best in rapidly dividing cells, whereas the effects in tumors with slower growth fractions and lower mitotic indices might be reduced [11]. Early stages of EMM are small and often extraordinary slow-growing [21]. Therefore, even if high concentrations of BA or NVX-207 had reached the centrally located cells within the solid tumors, these cells may have had a particularly slow replicative rate and were, in consequence, less sensitive to the compounds [11]. This could be another reason why the treated tumors reacted only slowly to the therapy. If a prospective improved pharmaceutical formulation could increase the penetration depth and concentration of the active ingredients in the tumors, an application in study horses suffering from larger, faster growing tumors would potentially be conceivable.

With regard to the *in vitro* and *in vivo* data about BA and NVX-207 reported here and previously [96,110,137], it seems surprising that NVX-207 had less *in vivo* anticancer effects on the melanocytic lesions than its parent BA. The determined *in vitro* IC_{50} concentrations for NVX-207 leading to antiproliferative and cytotoxic effects in EMM cells were much lower than those calculated for BA. Furthermore, the amount of NVX-207 found in the skin of healthy horses after topical application was considerably higher than the concentrations of BA. The tumor microenvironment of a solid tumor comprises the tumor cells themselves, but also resident and infiltrating nontumor cells like fibroblasts, endothelial cells, macrophages, other immune cells and the cytokines, chemokines, and growth factors that they secrete [174,175]. Hence, a reliable transferability of *in vitro* results gained from monolayer cell culture experiments with cancer cells to *in vivo* conditions is not always given and tumor cells in their native microenvironment can be much more robust against chemotherapeutic influences [172–174]. It is also conceivable that esterases in the skin have cleaved the active groups of NVX-207 at the C-3 and C-28 position, thus, rendering the substance ineffective or less effective [176]. Indeed, deacetyl-

TRIS, a decomposition product of NVX-207, was also investigated by the project partners of the Biozentrum (Martin-Luther-University Halle-Wittenberg) in cell culture experiments and tested as significantly less effective against EMM cells MelDuWi and other human cancer cells than NVX-207 (unpublished data). However, it is only speculative that a cleavage takes place and appropriate studies have to be carried out to clarify this hypothesis. If the latter proves to be true the next step would be to develop a drug carrier (i.e. liposome, microemulsion) that protects the active ingredient from enzymatic hydrolysis or oxidation, delivers it intact to the desired layer(s) in the skin and, hence, increases its bioavailability [85,177]. The results of the skin sample examinations by means of HPLC analysis from the permeation studies clearly verified the intact substance NVX-207 in healthy equine skin, which in turn speaks against this assumption. Although the generated *in vitro* data on NVX-207 showed greater promise than the results from the clinical efficacy trial, there were still valuable insights obtained with respect to the effective mode of action in equine skin cancer cells and the *in vivo* safety and efficacy of the compound. Nevertheless, the existing data fail to resolve the contradiction between *in vitro* cell culture experiments and *in vivo* efficacy study.

Even though no complete tumor regression was observed after 91 days of treatment, the preliminary observations from the efficacy study indicate that topical BA application might be a feasible treatment to successfully stabilize or even reduce tumor bulk in early stage EMM cases. This could, thus, reduce the health risks associated with the malignant degeneration of tumors. BA has been demonstrated to exert greater anticancer effects in an environment with a pH lower than 6.8 [178,179]. From a clinical perspective, this is an important property of the compound since microenvironmental acidification is found in the majority of tumors as a consequence of upregulated glycolysis and inadequate drainage through tumor tissue perfusion [180,181]. To the author's best knowledge, no data about pH values in EMM tissue exist. However, those in human melanoma have been reported to range from 6.4 to 7.3 [181]. There are no reports about the cytotoxicity of NVX-207 in an acidic microenvironment and reduced efficacy at low pH may explain why NVX-207 was less effective than BA in the present study. Investigations carried out by the project partner Skinomics GmbH showed that NVX-207 remains stable under acidic conditions to more than 94% (unpublished data). Further studies must follow to prove the effectiveness of the compound in equine cancer cells in an environment with acidic pH.

Although the topical treatment of early stages of EMM with 1 % BA and 1 % NVX-207 resulted in part in tumor volume reductions, the results should be interpreted against the background that two tumors (both horse 18) in the placebo group also showed a decrease in tumor size that matched the definition of response to therapy. Histopathological examinations of the treated skin at neck and ventral tail in study III revealed a perivascularly accentuated, lymphohistiocytic inflammation with few neutrophils in the superficial dermis. Results indicated that the activation of the immune system was associated with ingredients in the carrier cream "Basiscreme DAC", as the alterations were observed in the placebo group also. Hence, the repeated topical application of the study medication for 13 consecutive weeks in combination with the covering of the treatment sites could have led to an increased blood supply to the tumor area with increased immune cell infiltration not only in horses treated with BA and NVX-207, but also in horses treated with the placebo [182]. Tumor infiltrating lymphocytes are associated with a favorable prognostic role in the overall survival of human melanoma patients [183,184]. Unfortunately, no histopathological examinations of the treated melanomas with appropriate staining for vascularization markers or immune cell typing could be performed, because skin biopsy samplings were not accepted by the stud management. This can be considered a limitation of the present study. Thus, appropriate investigations are recommended for future studies in order to elucidate if immunological adjuvant effects are involved in the tumor volume reduction.

Study horse compliance. Even after 13 consecutive weeks of topical treatment twice a day the equine patient compliance was very good. On the one hand, the study horses were broodmares and therefore used to a manipulation in the sense of lifting the tail. On the other hand, neither the horses enrolled in the study described in manuscript III nor private horses, in which the tail was lifted for tests, showed defensive movements. The inconspicuous behavior of the mares may also indicate that the treatment did not cause painful inflammatory reactions in the skin. These observations are in line with the findings from study III demonstrating that mild clinical skin changes occurred dominantly in the skin of the neck rather than on the tail. Thus, the topical therapy of melanomas located on the ventral tail and in the perianal region has been proven to be very feasible in this study. On the contrary, the topical approach for melanomas located in the lip is probably not suitable due to the risk of the horse licking the cream and absorbing it orally.

Local and systemic safety. The regular physical examinations of the study horses were unremarkable and no clinically relevant abnormalities in serial blood samplings were noted. The mild colic diagnosed in two horses each could be associated with reasons other than the topical therapy. The follow-up examinations four month after the last treatment revealed that all horses enrolled in the study were healthy and the treated tumors were stable in size. The occasionally observed depigmentation of some EMM was a temporary side effect that had vanished by the time of the follow-up examination.

Efficacy study – Conclusion. To summarize, the observations from study IV indicate that the topical application of 1 % BA and 1 % NVX-207 over a period of 13 weeks is practicable and safe in horses. A greater number of tumors responded to the therapy with BA and NVX-207

than tumors from the placebo group. Furthermore, the non-invasiveness of the treatment and the good patient compliance have been extensively demonstrated. By using only horses of the same breed and sex, good comparisons could be made within the treatment groups and also between the groups. However, patient selection and small sample size of the current study clearly limits the conclusions for a more diverse and larger horse population. Consequently, large-scale studies are required to verify the preliminary results reported here.
Nevertheless, the long treatment period and the application twice a day is a disadvantage of the developed study medications as these could lead to a negligent treatment by the horse owners. Besides that, no complete tumor regression was observed in any of the tumors treated. Although the reported results indicate that the topical therapy may represent an alternative to the surgical excision or to the frequently practiced approach of benign neglect of small solitary masses, the aforementioned drawbacks emphasize the need for modifications in the current formulations or techniques to improve the skin penetration and permeation in skin affected by EMM. Prospective, modified formulations can certainly have a more "modern" and innovative composition than the one used in the current PhD project. The cutaneous delivery of anticancer drugs can be improved either by increasing drug solubility in the *stratum corneum*, by increasing drug diffusivity in the skin and tumor tissue, or by increasing the degree of saturation of the drug in the formulation [185]. Thus, the antitumor effects of the compounds may be favorably influenced by a dose increase of BA and NVX-207 in the test formulation. Future studies could further focus on other modifications in the topical applied vehicle, such as the incorporation of permeation enhancers that transport large amounts of the active ingredient through the fibrous tumor capsule of EMM to the tumor cells [85]. Besides, nanocarrier systems like liposomes [71,85] and microemulsions [177,186] are well known examples of delivery vehicles or carriers for hydrophobic drugs.

Despite significant understanding of the pathogenesis, risk factors and diagnosis of human cutaneous melanoma, this disease is responsible for the vast majority of skin cancer-related deaths in the fair-skinned population [187]. Since grey horses suffering from EMM are repeatedly discussed and used as a translational research model for human melanoma [20,36,50,55,188,189], the combined results of the four studies presented herein could also be useful for human medical research. The compounds investigated in this thesis have been reported to exert a good cytotoxic and apoptotic efficacy in human melanoma cells, as shown for BA in human melanoma cell lines MEL-1, -2, -3, -4 [113], Mel-Juso [190], MeWo [156], 518A2 [150], and A375 [96,150] and NVX-207 in human melanoma cell lines 518A2 [137] and A375 [96]. Consequently, an adaptation of the results to human applications is possible, especially if subsequent projects to this PhD project also progress positively. If the latter proves to be true, there is a real possibility of arousing the interest of larger veterinary or human pharmaceutical companies in the further development of the topical drug. This assumption is supported by the fact that two studies have already been carried out on the topical application of BA in human patients suffering from dysplastic melanocytic nevus and cutaneous metastatic melanoma [98,191]. Unfortunately, study results from the clinical trials have not been published so far. Summarized, the increasing interest in triterpenes and their derivatives [148] together with the results demonstrated in this thesis may well stimulate the search for a safe and effective drug for use in cutaneous cancers of diverse histological types in animal and human patients.

7. Major findings and conclusions

The experiments conducted within the framework of the current thesis provide an important contribution to the development of a topical drug against EMM and ES. A strength of the present work is that in addition to numerous *in vitro* experiments, studies have also been carried out on the target species, thus enabling a direct comparison of the generated data. The triterpene BA, its derivative NVX-207 and the betulin derivative BBS were demonstrated to exert significant antiproliferative and cytotoxic effects in primary EMM, primary ES cells and primary equine dermal fibroblasts. Importantly, these *in vitro* anticancer effects were shown to be triggered by the induction of apoptosis. Further, new insights into the *in vitro* penetration and permeation profiles of BA and NVX-207 in isolated equine skin were given. In accordance with these results, the amounts of BA and NVX-207 detected by HPLC in horse skin *in vivo* exceeded by far the previously determined IC_{50} values of EMM and ES cells. In this context, the local and systemic safety of BA and NVX-207 applied topically were proven. Even though no complete remission of the tumors could be achieved with the investigated pharmaceutical formulations in early stage EMM, a clear tumor response was observed after treatment with both BA and NVX-207. The findings of the efficacy study must be regarded as preliminary due to the limited group size and need to be replicated in a larger cohort. Prospective studies should primarily focus on the modification of the pharmaceutical formulation in order to further improve the clinical outcome. Taken together, the discussed studies of this PhD project provide valuable pieces in a big puzzle which – when complete – could lead to an effective, marketable topical drug which reduces health risks associated with EMM and ES and, consequently, improve the welfare of equine skin cancer patients.

8. Future perspectives

The efficacy and active mode of action of BA and NVX-207 in EMM and ES cells have already been proven by previous research [96] as well as cell culture experiments reported here. Concentration profiles for both compounds were investigated in normal equine skin *in vitro* and *in vivo*. Altered concentration profiles of BA and NVX-207 in tumor-affected skin may have limited the efficacy of the substances in the clinical trial reported in manuscript IV. "Just as it's easier to carry a drink in a glass rather than on a plate, finding the right carrier for medications helps to ensure they arrive at their destination intact" [192]. Therefore, future research projects should focus on the modification of the pharmaceutical formulations.

Different approaches exist to further improve the *stratum corneum* penetration and increase skin permeability in order to reach the full depth of tumor invasion with sufficiently high concentrations of the active substance. An enhanced drug diffusivity in the skin could be achieved by disordering the *stratum corneum* lipids with chemical penetration enhancers like DMSO [193] or oleic acid [194]. Propylene glycol and diethylene glycol monoethyl ether are drugs, which are thought to increase drug solubility in the skin [185]. The cutaneous delivery of BA or NVX-207 could further be improved by increasing the degree of saturation of the drugs in the formulation [185]. Vasoconstrictor substances incorporated into the carrier vehicle could influence drug absorption in the dermis and lead to enhanced local concentrations of the compounds [195]. Incorporation of nanocarrier systems like liposomes [71], polymeric and lipid nanoparticles [85] and microemulsions [186] could be other approaches that include advantages like low potential for skin irritation, increased protection of the encapsulated drug, and penetration-enhancing properties.

Prospective *in vitro* trials should be conducted not only on unaltered, but also on skin affected by EMM or ES – even if a standardized procedure is difficult to achieve with tumor skin. Only in this way, the influence on the permeation of possibly existing tumor-induced skin changes such as ulcerations, hyperplasia of the epidermis or fibrotic tumor capsules as well as the permeation in the tumor tissue itself can be assessed directly. In addition, besides FDC cell experiments, even more sensitive and sophisticated techniques like cutaneous microdialysis [87] or confocal laser scanning microscopy [196] could be applied.

Furthermore, combinational therapies with BA, NVX-207, BBS, or other triterpenoids or protocols combining the phytochemical treatment with surgery or radiotherapy could be considered for future studies to enhance the antitumor efficacy. To gain reliable data on the efficacy of the topically applied drugs in equine patients suffering from EMM and/or ES, further longitudinal, placebo-controlled, randomized, blinded large-scale trials in a multi-centric approach with long-term follow-ups should be performed.

9. References

[1] Baker JR, Leyland A. Histological survey of tumours of the horse, with particular reference to those of the skin. Vet Rec 1975;96:419–22.

[2] Scott DW, Miller WH. Equine Dermatology. 2nd ed. Maryland Heights: Elsevier Saunders; 2011.

[3] Valentine BA. Survey of equine cutaneous neoplasia in the Pacific Northwest. J Vet Diagnostics Investig 2006;18:123–6.

[4] Johnson PJ. Dermatologic tumors (excluding sarcoids). Vet Clin North Am Equine Pract 1998;14:625–58. https://doi.org/10.1016/S0749-0739(17)30190-6.

[5] Marti E, Lazary S, Antczak DF, Gerber H. Report of the first international workshop on equine sarcoid. Equine Vet J 1993;25:397–407. https://doi.org/10.1111/j.2042-3306.1993.tb02981.x.

[6] Nasir L, Brandt S. Papillomavirus associated diseases of the horse. Vet Microbiol 2013;167:159–67. https://doi.org/10.1016/j.vetmic.2013.08.003.

[7] Macgillivray KC, Sweeney RW, Piero F Del. Metastatic Melanoma in Horses. J Vet Intern Med 2002;16:452–6.

[8] Wang XJ, Chen JY, Fu LQ, Yan MJ. Recent advances in natural therapeutic approaches for the treatment of cancer. J Chemother 2020;32:53–65. https://doi.org/10.1080/1120009X.2019.1707417.

[9] Amaral RG, Santos SA dos, Andrade LN, Severino P, Carvalho AA. Natural Products as Treatment against Cancer: A Historical and Current Vision. Clin Oncol 2019;4:1–5.

[10] Reed S, Bayly WM, Sellon D. Equine Internal Medicine. St. Louis, Missouri: Elsevier Inc; 4th ed. 2018.

[11] Knottenbelt DC, Patterson-Kane JC, Snalune KL. Clinical Equine Oncology. St. Louis, Missouri: Elsevier Ltd; 2015. https://doi.org/10.1016/c2009-0-61955-3.

[12] Sundberg JP, Burnstein T, Page EH, Kirkham WW RF. Neoplasms of Equidae. J Am Vet Med Assoc 1997;170:150–2. https://doi.org/10.137.

[13] Knowles EJ, Tremaine WH, Pearson GR, Mair TS. A database survey of equine tumours in the United Kingdom. Equine Vet J 2016;48:280–4. https://doi.org/10.1111/evj.12421.

[14] Seltenhammer MH, Simhofer H, Scherzer S, Zechner P, Curik I, Sölkner J, et al. Equine melanoma in a population of 296 grey Lipizzaner horses. Equine Vet J 2003;35:153–7. https://doi.org/10.2746/042516403776114234.

[15] Fleury C, Bérard F, Balme B, Thomas L. The study of cutaneous melanomas in Camargue-type gray-skinned horses (1): Clinical pathological characterization. Pigment Cell Res 2000;13:39–46. https://doi.org/10.1034/j.1600-0749.2000.130108.x.

[16] McFadyean J. Equine melanomatosis. J Comp Pathol Ther 1933;46:186–204. https://doi.org/http://dx.doi.org/10.1016/S0368-1742(33)80025-7.

[17] Valentine BA. Equine Melanocytic Tumors: A Retrospective Study of 53 Horses (1988 to 1991). J Vet Intern Med 1995;9:291–7. https://doi.org/10.1111/j.1939-1676.1995.tb01087.x.

[18] Phillips JC, Lembcke LM. Equine melanocytic tumors. Vet Clin North Am - Equine Pract 2013;29:673–87. https://doi.org/10.1016/j.cveq.2013.08.008.

[19] Smith SH, Goldschmidt MH, McManus PM. A Comparative Review of Melanocytic Neoplasms. Vet Pathol 2002;39:651–78.

[20] Seltenhammer MH, Heere-Ress E, Brandt S, Druml T, Jansen B, Pehamberger H, et al. Comparative histopathology of grey-horse-melanoma and human malignant melanoma. Pigment Cell Res 2004;17:674–81. https://doi.org/10.1111/j.1600-0749.2004.00192.x.

[21] Moore JS, Shaw C, Shaw E, Buechner-Maxwell V, Scarratt WK, Crisman M, et al. Melanoma in horses: Current perspectives. Equine Vet Educ 2013;25:144–51. https://doi.org/10.1111/j.2042-3292.2011.00368.x.

[22] MacKay RJ. Treatment Options for Melanoma of Gray Horses. Vet Clin North Am - Equine Pract 2019;35:311–25. https://doi.org/10.1016/j.cveq.2019.04.003.

[23] Rosengren Pielberg G, Golovko A, Sundström E, Curik I, Lennartsson J, Seltenhammer MH, et al. A cis-acting regulatory mutation causes premature hair graying and susceptibility to melanoma in the horse. Nat Genet 2008;40:1004–9. https://doi.org/10.1038/ng.185.

[24] Curik I, Druml T, Seltenhammer M, Sundström E, Pielberg GR, Andersson L, et al. Complex Inheritance of Melanoma and Pigmentation of Coat and Skin in Grey Horses. PLoS Genet 2013; 40:1004–9. https://doi.org/10.1371/journal.pgen.1003248.

[25] Sánchez-Guerrero MJ, Solé M, Azor PJ, Sölkner J, Valera M. Genetic and environmental risk factors for vitiligo and melanoma in Pura Raza Español horses. Equine Vet J 2019;51:606–11. https://doi.org/10.1111/evj.13067.

[26] Sundström E, Imsland F, Mikko S, Wade C, Sigurdsson S, Pielberg G, et al. Copy number expansion of the STX17 duplication in melanoma tissue from Grey horses. BMC Genomics 2012; 13:1–13. https://doi.org/10.1186/1471-2164-13-365.

[27] Bastian BC. The Molecular Pathology of Melanoma: An Integrated Taxonomy of Melanocytic Neoplasia. vol. 9. 2014. https://doi.org/10.1146/annurev-pathol-012513-104658.

[28] Sundström E, Komisarczuk AZ, Jiang L, Golovko A, Navratilova P, Rinkwitz S, et al. Identification of a melanocyte-specific, microphthalmia-associated transcription factor-dependent regulatory element in the intronic duplication causing hair greying and melanoma in horses. Pigment Cell Melanoma Res 2012;25:28–36. https://doi.org/10.1111/j.1755-148X.2011.00902.x.

[29] Dixon J, Smith K, Perkins J, Sherlock C, Mair T, Weller R. Computed tomographic appearance of melanomas in the equine head: 13 cases. Vet Radiol Ultrasound 2016;57:246–52. https://doi.org/10.1111/vru.12345.

[30] Cavalleri J V, Mählmann K, Steinig P, Feige K. Aetiology , clinical presentation and current treatment options of equine malignant melanoma – a review of the literature. Pferdeheilkunde 2014;30:455–60. https://doi.org/10.21836/PEM20140410.

[31] Scott D. Neoplastic Diseases. In: Pedersen D, editor. Large Anim. Dermatology, Philadelphia, USA: W.B. Saunders Company; 1988, p. 448–52.

[32] Strauss RA, Allbaugh RA, Haynes J, Ben-Shlomo G. Primary corneal malignant melanoma in a horse. Equine Vet Educ 2017:1–7. https://doi.org/10.1111/eve.12815.

[33] Caston SS, Fales-Williams A. Primary malignant melanoma in the oesophagus of a foal. Equine Vet Educ 2010;22:387–90. https://doi.org/doi:10.1111/j.2042-3292.2010.00050.x.

[34] Kovac M, Ueberschär S, Nowak M, Prange T, Mundt-Wüstenberg S. Aortic valve insufficiency and myocardial melanoma in a horse. Pferdeheilkd Equine Med 2005;21:408–12. https://doi.org/10.21836/PEM20050502.

[35] Rodríguez F, Forga J, Herráez P, Andrada M, Fernández A. Metastatic melanoma causing spinal cord compression in a horse. Vet Rec 1998;142:248–9. https://doi.org/10.1136/vr.142.10.248.

[36] Campagne C, Julé S, Bernex F, Estrada M, Aubin-Houzelstein G, Panthier JJ, et al. RACK1, a clue to the diagnosis of cutaneous melanomas in horses. BMC Vet Res 2012;8:1–9. https://doi.org/10.1186/1746-6148-8-95.

[37] Balch CM, Buzaid AC, Soong S-J, Atkins MB, Cascinelli N, Coit DG, et al. Final Version of the American Joint Committee on Cancer Staging System for Cutaneous Melanoma. J Clin Oncol 2001;19:3635–48.

[38] Covington AL, Magdesian KG, Madigan JE, Maleski K, Gray LC, Smith PA, et al. Recurrent Esophageal Obstruction and Dysphagia due to a Brainstem Melanoma in a Horse. J Vet Intern Med 2004;18:245–7. https://doi.org/10.1892/0891-6640(2004)18<245:REOADD>2.0.CO;2.

[39] Patterson-Kane JC, Sanchez LC, Uhl EW, Edens LM. Disseminated metastatic intramedullary melanoma in an aged grey horse. J Comp Pathol 2001;125:204–7. https://doi.org/10.1053/jcpa.2001.0481.

[40] Milne JC. Malignant melanomas causing Horner's syndrome in a horse. Equine Vet J 1986;18:74–5. https://doi.org/doi:10.1111/j.2042-3306.1986.tb03545.x.

[41] Groom LM, Sullins KE. Surgical excision of large melanocytic tumours in grey horses: 38 cases (2001–2013). Equine Vet Educ 2018;30:438–43. https://doi.org/10.1111/eve.12767.

[42] Rowe EL, Sullins KE. Excision as treatment of dermal melanomatosis in horses: 11 cases (1994-2000). J

Am Vet Med Assoc 2004;225:94–6. https://doi.org/10.2460/javma.2004.225.94.

[43] Goetz TE, Ogilvie GK, Keegan KG, Johnson PJ. Cimetidine for treatment of melanomas in three horses. J Am Vet Med Assoc 1990;196:449–52.

[44] Laus F, Cerquetella M, Paggi E, Ippedico G, Argentieri M, Castellano G, et al. Evaluation of cimetidine as a therapy for dermal melanomatosis in grey horse. Isr J Vet Med 2010;65:47–52.

[45] Théon AP, Wilson WD, Magdesian KG, Pusterla N, Snyder JR, Galuppo LD. Long-term outcome associated with intratumoral chemotherapy with cisplatin for cutaneous tumors in equidae: 573 cases (1995-2004). J Am Vet Med Assoc 2007;230:1506–13. https://doi.org/10.2460/javma.230.10.1506.

[46] Spugnini EP, D'Alterio GL, Dotsinsky I, Mudrov T, Dragonetti E, Murace R, et al. Electrochemotherapy for the Treatment of Multiple Melanomas in a Horse. J Equine Vet Sci 2011;31:430–3. https://doi.org/10.1016/j.jevs.2011.01.009.

[47] Hewes C a, Sullins KE. Use of cisplatin-containing biodegradable beads for treatment of cutaneous neoplasia in equidae: 59 cases (2000-2004). J Am Vet Med Assoc 2006;229:1617–22. https://doi.org/10.2460/javma.229.10.1617.

[48] Heinzerling LM, Feige K, Rieder S, Akens MK, Dummer R, Stranzinger G, et al. Tumor regression induced by intratumoral injection of DNA coding for human interleukin 12 into melanoma metastases in gray horses. J Mol Med 2000;78:692–702. https://doi.org/10.1007/s001090000165.

[49] Mählmann K, Feige K, Juhls C, Endmann A, Schuberth H-J, Oswald D, et al. Local and systemic effect of transfection-reagent formulated DNA vectors on equine melanoma. BMC Vet Res 2015;11:1–11. https://doi.org/10.1186/s12917-015-0422-9.

[50] Müller JMV, Feige K, Wunderlin P, Hödl A, Meli ML, Seltenhammer M, et al. Double-blind placebo-controlled study with interleukin-18 and interleukin-12-encoding plasmid DNA shows antitumor effect in metastatic melanoma in gray horses. J Immunother 2011;34:58–64. https://doi.org/10.1097/CJI.0b013e3181fe1997.

[51] Bradley WM, Schilpp D, Khatibzadeh SM. Electronic brachytherapy used for the successful treatment of three different types of equine tumours. Equine Vet Educ 2017;29:293–8. https://doi.org/10.1111/eve.12420.

[52] Henson FMD, Dobson JM. Use of radiation therapy in the treatment of equine neoplasia. Equine Vet Educ 2010;16:315–8. https://doi.org/10.1111/j.2042-3292.2004.tb00319.x.

[53] Sanderson BJS, Ferguson LR, Denny WA. Mutagenic and carcinogenic properties of platinum-based anticancer drugs. Mutat Res - Fundam Mol Mech Mutagen 1996;355:59–70. https://doi.org/10.1016/0027-5107(96)00022-X.

[54] Soe L, Wurz GT, Mäenpää JU, Hubbard GB, Cadman TB, Wiebe VJ, et al. Tissue distribution of transdermal toremifene. Cancer Chemother Pharmacol 1997;39:513–20. https://doi.org/10.1007/s002800050607.

[55] Moore JS. A Translational Study Evaluating the Uses of Diagnostic and Therapeutic Practices Established in Human Malignant Melanoma in Equine Malignant Melanoma [Doctoral dissertation]. Virginia Polytechnic Institute and State University, 2013.

[56] Goodrich L, Gerber H, Marti E, Antczak DF. Equine sarcoids. Vet Clin North Am Equine Pract 1998;14:607–23. https://doi.org/10.1016/S0749-0739(17)30189-X.

[57] Taylor S, Haldorson G. A review of equine sarcoid. Equine Vet Educ 2013;25:210–6. https://doi.org/doi: 10.1111/j.2042-3292.2012.00411.x.

[58] Hainisch EK, Brandt S. Equine Sarcoid. Robinson's Current Therapy in Equine Medicine. Seventh Ed. Elsevier Inc.; 2014. https://doi.org/10.1016/B978-1-4557-4555-5.00099-6.

[59] Knottenbelt DC. A suggested clinical classification for the equine sarcoid. Clin Tech Equine Pract 2005;4:278–95. https://doi.org/10.1053/j.ctep.2005.10.008.

[60] Chambers G, Ellsmore VA, O'Brien PM, Reid SWJ, Love S, Campo MS, et al. Association of bovine papillomavirus with the equine sarcoid. J Gen Virol 2003;84:1055–62. https://doi.org/10.1099/vir.0.18947-0.

[61] Yuan ZQ, Gault EA, Saveria Campo M, Nasir L. Different contribution of bovine papillomavirus type 1 oncoproteins to the transformation of equine fibroblasts. J Gen Virol 2011;92:773–83.

https://doi.org/10.1099/vir.0.028191-0.

[62] Martens A, De Moor A, Ducatelle R. PCR Detection of Bovine Papilloma Virus DNA in Superficial Swabs and Scrapings from Equine Sarcoids. Vet J 2001;161:280–6. https://doi.org/10.1053/tvjl.2000.0524.

[63] Staiger EA, Tseng CT, Miller D, Cassano JM, Nasir L, Garrick D, et al. Host genetic influence on papillomavirus-induced tumors in the horse. Int J Cancer 2016;139:784–92. https://doi.org/10.1002/ijc.30120.

[64] Angelos J, Oppenheim Y, Rebhun W, Mohammed H, Antczak DF. Evaluation of breed as a risk factor for sarcoid and uveitis in horses. Anim Genet 1988;19:417–25. https://doi.org/10.1111/j.1365-2052.1988.tb00833.x.

[65] Martens A, De Moor A, Demeulemeester J, Ducatelle R. Histopathological characteristics of five clinical types of equine sarcoid. Res Vet Sci 2000. https://doi.org/10.1053/rvsc.2000.0432.

[66] Compston PC, Turner T, Wylie CE, Payne RJ. Laser surgery as a treatment for histologically confirmed sarcoids in the horse. Equine Vet J 2016;48:451–6. https://doi.org/10.1111/evj.12456.

[67] Carstanjen B, Jordan P, Lepage OM. Carbon dioxide laser as a surgical instrument for sarcoid therapy - A retrospective study on 60 cases. Can Vet Journal-Revue Vet Can 1997;38:773–6.

[68] Haspeslagh M, Vlaminck LEM, Martens AM. Treatment of sarcoids in equids: 230 cases (2008–2013). J Am Vet Med Assoc 2016;249:311–8. https://doi.org/10.2460/javma.249.3.311.

[69] Stadler S, Kainzbauer C, Haralambus R, Brehm W, Hainisch E, Brandt S. Successful treatment of equine sarcoids by topical aciclovir application. Vet Rec 2011;168:1–4. https://doi.org/10.1136/vr.c5430.

[70] Knottenbelt DC, Walker JA. Topical treatment of the equine sarcoid. Equine Vet Educ 1994;6:72–5.

[71] Knottenbelt DC, Watson AH, Hotchkiss JW, Chopra S, Higgins AJ. A pilot study on the use of ultra-deformable liposomes containing bleomycin in the treatment of equine sarcoid. Equine Vet Educ 2018;32:258–63. https://doi.org/10.1111/eve.12950.

[72] Tozon N, Kramaric P, Kos Kadunc V, Sersa G, Cemazar M. Electrochemotherapy as a single or adjuvant treatment to surgery of cutaneous sarcoid tumours in horses: A 31-case retrospective study. Vet Rec 2016;179:1–5. https://doi.org/10.1136/vr.103867.

[73] Martens A, De Moor A, Vlaminck L, Pille F, Steenhaut M. Evaluation of excision, cryosurgery and local BCG vaccination for the treatment of equine sarcoids. Vet Rec 2001;149:665–9. https://doi.org/10.1136/vr.149.22.665.

[74] Rothacker CC, Boyle AG, Levine DG. Autologous vaccination for the treatment of equine sarcoids: 18 cases(2009-2014). Can Vet J 2015; 56:709–714.

[75] Vanselow BA, Abetz I, Jackson AR. BCG emulsion immunotherapy of equine sarcoid. Equine Vet J 1988;20:444–7. https://doi.org/10.1111/j.2042-3306.1988.tb01571.x.

[76] Hainisch EK, Abel-Reichwald H, Shafti-Keramat S, Pratscher B, Corteggio A, Borzacchiello G, et al. Potential of a BPV1 L1 VLP vaccine to prevent BPV1- or BPV2- induced pseudo-sarcoid formation and safety and immunogenicity of EcPV2 L1 VLPs in horse. J Gen Virol 2017;98:230–41. https://doi.org/10.1099/jgv.0.000673.

[77] Hollis AR. Strontium plesiotherapy for the treatment of sarcoids in the horse. Equine Vet Educ 2020;32:7–11. https://doi.org/10.1111/eve.13038.

[78] Byam-Cook KL, Henson FMD, Slater JD. Treatment of periocular and non-ocular sarcoids in 18 horses by interstitial brachytherapy with iridium-192. Vet Rec 2006;159:337–41. https://doi.org/10.1136/vr.159.11.337.

[79] Théon AP, Pascoe JR. Iridium-192 interstitial brachytherapy for equine periocular tumours: treatment results and prognostic factors in 115 horses. Equine Vet J 1995;27:117–21. https://doi.org/doi:10.1111/j.2042-3306.1995.tb03046.x.

[80] Golding JP, Kemp-Symonds JG, Dobson JM. Glycolysis inhibition improves photodynamic therapy response rates for equine sarcoids. Vet Comp Oncol 2017;15:1543–52. https://doi.org/10.1111/vco.12299.

[81] Martens A, Moor ADE, Waelkens E, Merlevede W, De Witte P. In vitro and in vivo evaluation of hypericin for photodynamic therapy of equine sarcoids. Vet J 2000;159:77–84.

https://doi.org/10.1053/tvjl.1999.0392.

[82] Christen-Clottu O, Klocke P, Burger D, Straub R, Gerber V. Treatment of Clinically Diagnosed Equine Sarcoid with a Mistletoe Extract (Viscum album austriacus). J Vet Intern Med 2010;24:1483–9. https://doi.org/10.1111/j.1939-1676.2010.0597.x.

[83] Wilford S, Woodward E, Dunkel B. Owners' perception of the efficacy of Newmarket bloodroot ointment in treating equine sarcoids. Can Vet J 2014;55:683–6.

[84] Knottenbelt DC. The Equine Sarcoid: Why Are There so Many Treatment Options? Vet Clin North Am - Equine Pract 2019;35:243–62. https://doi.org/10.1016/j.cveq.2019.03.006.

[85] Fleury S, Vianna Lopez RF. Topical Administration of Anticancer Drugs for Skin Cancer Treatment. In: Caterina AM La Porta, editor. Ski. Cancers - Risk Factors, Prev. Ther., IntechOpen; 2011, p. 247–72. https://doi.org/10.5772/27785.

[86] Haspeslagh M, Jordana Garcia M, Vlaminck LEM, Martens AM. Topical use of 5% acyclovir cream for the treatment of occult and verrucous equine sarcoids: A double-blinded placebo-controlled study. BMC Vet Res 2017;13:1–6. https://doi.org/10.1186/s12917-017-1215-0.

[87] Luís A, Ruela M, Perissinato AG, Esselin M, Lino DS. Evaluation of skin absorption of drugs from topical and transdermal formulations. Brazilian J Pharm Sci 2016;52:527–44. https://doi.org/http://dx.doi.org/10.1590/S1984-82502016000300018.

[88] Bouwstra JA, Ponec M. The skin barrier in healthy and diseased state. Biochim Biophys Acta - Biomembr 2006;1758:2080–95. https://doi.org/10.1016/j.bbamem.2006.06.021.

[89] Stahl J, Niedorf F, Kietzmann M. Characterisation of epidermal lipid composition and skin morphology of animal skin ex vivo. Eur J Pharm Biopharm 2009;72:310–6. https://doi.org/10.1016/j.ejpb.2008.09.013.

[90] Prausnitz MR, Elias PM, Franz TJ, Schmuth M, Tsai J-C, Menon GK, et al. Skin Barrier and Transdermal Drug Delivery. Med Ther 2012;5:2065–73.

[91] Kalia YN, Guy RH. Modeling transdermal drug release. Adv Drug Deliv Rev 2001;48:159–72. https://doi.org/10.1016/S0169-409X(01)00113-2.

[92] Mohd F, Todo H, Yoshimoto M, Yusuf E, Sugibayashi K. Contribution of the hair follicular pathway to total skin permeation of topically applied and exposed chemicals. Pharmaceutics 2016;8:1–12. https://doi.org/10.3390/pharmaceutics8040032.

[93] Stahl J, Kietzmann M. The effects of chemical and physical penetration enhancers on the percutaneous permeation of lidocaine through equine skin. BMC Vet Res 2014;10:1–6. https://doi.org/10.1186/1746-6148-10-138.

[94] OECD/OCDE. OECD Guideline for the testing of chemicals No. 428: Skin Absorption: in vitro Method. France: 2004. https://doi.org/https://doi.org/10.1787/20745788.

[95] OECD. Guidance Document for the Conduct of Skin Absorption Studies. OECD Environmental Health and Safety Publications Series on Testing and Assessment No. 28. France: 2004. https://doi.org/https://doi.org/10.1787/9789264078796-en.

[96] Liebscher G, Vanchangiri K, Mueller T, Feige K, Cavalleri JMV, Paschke R. In vitro anticancer activity of Betulinic acid and derivatives thereof on equine melanoma cell lines from grey horses and invivo safety assessment of the compound NVX-207 in two horses. Chem Biol Interact 2016;246:20–9. https://doi.org/10.1016/j.cbi.2016.01.002.

[97] Xu R, Fazio GC, Matsuda SPT. On the origins of triterpenoid skeletal diversity. Phytochemistry 2004;65:261–91. https://doi.org/10.1016/j.phytochem.2003.11.014.

[98] Zalesińska MD, Borska S. Betulin and its derivatives – precursors of new drugs. World Sci News 2019;127:123–38.

[99] Oliveira Costa JF, Barbosa-Filho JM, De Azevedo Maia GL, Guimarães ET, Meira CS, Ribeiro-Dos-Santos R, et al. Potent anti-inflammatory activity of betulinic acid treatment in a model of lethal endotoxemia. Int Immunopharmacol 2014;23:469–74. https://doi.org/10.1016/j.intimp.2014.09.021.

[100] Del Carmen Recio M, Giner RM, Manez S, Gueho J, Julien HR, Hostettmann K, et al. Investigations on the steroidal anti-inflammatory activity of triterpenoids from Diospyros leucomelas. Planta Med 1995;61:9–12. https://doi.org/10.1055/s-2006-957988.

[101] Laavola M, Haavikko R, Hämäläinen M, Leppänen T, Nieminen R, Alakurtti S, et al. Betulin Derivatives Effectively Suppress Inflammation in Vitro and in Vivo. J Nat Prod 2016;79:274–80. https://doi.org/10.1021/acs.jnatprod.5b00709.

[102] Haque S, Nawrot DA, Alakurtti S, Ghemtio L, Yli-Kauhaluoma J, Tammela P. Screening and characterisation of antimicrobial properties of semisynthetic betulin derivatives. PLoS One 2014;9:1–9. https://doi.org/10.1371/journal.pone.0102696.

[103] Schühly W, Heilmann J, Çalis I, Sticher O. New triterpenoids with antibacterial activity from Zizyphus joazeiro. Planta Med 1999;65:740–3. https://doi.org/10.1055/s-1999-14054.

[104] Enwerem NM, Okogun JI, Wambebe CO, Okorie DA, Akah PA. Anthelmintic activity of the stem bark extracts of Berlina grandiflora and one of its active principles, betulinic acid. Phytomedicine 2001;8:112–4. https://doi.org/10.1078/0944-7113-00023.

[105] Smith PF, Ogundele A, Forrest A, Wilton J, Salzwedel K, Doto J, et al. Phase I and II study of the safety, virologic effect, and pharmacokinetics/pharmacodynamics of single-dose 3-O-(3′3′-dimethylsuccinyl)betulinic acid (bevirimat) against human immunodeficiency virus Infection. Antimicrob Agents Chemother 2007;51:3574–81. https://doi.org/10.1128/AAC.00152-07.

[106] Fujioka T, Kashiwada Y, Kilkuskie RE, Cosentino LM, Bailas LM, Jiang JB, et al. Betulinic acid and platanic acid as anti-HIV principles from syzigium claviflorum, and the anti-HIV activity of structurally related triterpenoids. J Nat Prod 1994;57:243–7. https://doi.org/10.1111/j.1469-8986.1964.tb03225.x.

[107] Frew Q, Rennekampff H-O, Dziewulski P, Moiemen N, Zahn T, Hartmann B. Betulin wound gel accelerated healing of superficial partial thickness burns: Results of a randomized, intra-individually controlled, phase III trial with 12-months follow-up. Burns 2019;45:876–90. https://doi.org/10.1016/j.burns.2018.10.019.

[108] Yogeeswari P, Sriram D. Betulinic Acid and Its Derivatives: A Review on their Biological Properties. Curr Med Chem 2005;12:657–66. https://doi.org/10.2174/0929867053202214.

[109] Sarek J, Kvasnica M, Vlk M, Urban M, Dzubak P, Hajduch M. The Potential of Triterpenoids in the Treatment of Melanoma, Research on Melanoma - A Glimpse into Current Directions and Future Trends. Rijeka, Croatia: InTech; 2011. https://doi.org/http://dx.doi.org/10.5772/57353.

[110] Csuk R. Betulinic acid and its derivatives: a patent review (2008 – 2013). Expert Opin Ther Pat 2014;24:913–23. https://doi.org/10.1517/13543776.2014.927441.

[111] Plánder S, Simon B, Béni S, Alberti Á, Kéry Á, Székely E. Identification of triterpenes and β-sitosterol in the bark of plane tree extracts. Period Polytech Chem Eng 2019;63:340–7. https://doi.org/10.3311/PPch.12874.

[112] Csuk R, Schmuck K, Schäfer R. A practical synthesis of betulinic acid. Tetrahedron Lett 2006;47:8769–70. https://doi.org/10.1016/j.tetlet.2006.10.004.

[113] Pisha E, Chai H, Lee I-S, Chagwedera TE, Farnsworth NHS, Cordell GA, et al. Discovery of betulinic acid as a selective inhibitor of human melanoma that functions by induction of apoptosis. Nat Med 1995;1:1046–51. https://doi.org/10.1038/nm1095-1046.

[114] Ali-Seyed M, Jantan I, Vijayaraghavan K, Bukhari SNA. Betulinic Acid: Recent Advances in Chemical Modifications, Effective Delivery, and Molecular Mechanisms of a Promising Anticancer Therapy. Chem Biol Drug Des 2016;87:517–36. https://doi.org/10.1111/cbdd.12682.

[115] Fulda S, Friesen C, Los M, Scaffidi C, Mier W, Benedict M, et al. Betulinic acid triggers CD95 (APO-1/Fas)- and p53-independent apoptosis via activation of caspases in neuroectodermal tumors. Cancer Res 1997;57:4956–64.

[116] Rzeski W, Stepulak A, Szymański M, Sifringer M, Kaczor J, Wejksza K, et al. Betulinic acid decreases expression of bcl-2 and cyclin D1, inhibits proliferation, migration and induces apoptosis in cancer cells. Naunyn Schmiedebergs Arch Pharmacol 2006;374:11–20. https://doi.org/10.1007/s00210-006-0090-1.

[117] Soica C, Danciu C, Savoiu-Balint G, Borcan F, Ambrus R, Zupko I, et al. Betulinic acid in complex with a gamma-cyclodextrin derivative decreases proliferation and in vivo tumor development of non-metastatic and metastatic B164A5 cells. Int J Mol Sci 2014;15:8235–55. https://doi.org/10.3390/ijms15058235.

[118] Zhang X, Hu J, Chen Y. Betulinic acid and the pharmacological effects of tumor suppression (Review). Mol Med Rep 2016;14:4489–95. https://doi.org/10.3892/mmr.2016.5792.

[119] Zuco V, Supino R, Righetti SC, Cleris L, Marchesi E, Gambacorti-Passerini C, et al. Selective cytotoxicity of betulinic acid on tumor cell lines, but not on normal cells. Cancer Lett 2002;175:17–25. https://doi.org/10.1016/S0304-3835(01)00718-2.

[120] Kommera H, Kaluderović GN, Kalbitz J, Paschke R. Lupane Triterpenoids-Betulin and Betulinic acid derivatives induce apoptosis in tumor cells. Invest New Drugs 2011;29:266–72. https://doi.org/10.1007/s10637-009-9358-x.

[121] Wang P, Li Q, Li K, Zhang X, Han Z, Wang J, et al. Betulinic acid exerts immunoregulation and anti-tumor effect on cervical carcinoma (U14) tumor-bearing mice. Pharmazie 2012;67:733–9. https://doi.org/10.1691/ph.2012.1822.

[122] Wang W, Wang Y, Liu M, Zhang Y, Yang T, Li D, et al. Betulinic acid induces apoptosis and suppresses metastasis in hepatocellular carcinoma cell lines in vitro and in vivo. J Cell Mol Med 2018:1–10. https://doi.org/10.1111/jcmm.13964.

[123] Fulda S, Kroemer G. Targeting mitochondrial apoptosis by betulinic acid in human cancers. Drug Discov Today 2009;14:885–90. https://doi.org/10.1016/j.drudis.2009.05.015.

[124] Fulda S, Scaffidi G, Susin SA, Krammer PH, Kroemer G, Peter ME, et al. Activation of mitochondria and release of mitochondrial apoptogenic factors by betulinic acid. J Biol Chem 1998;273:33942–8. https://doi.org/10.1074/jbc.273.51.33942.

[125] Mullauer FB, Kessler JH, Medema JP. Betulinic acid induces cytochrome c release and apoptosis in a Bax/Bak-independent, permeability transition pore dependent fashion. Apoptosis 2009;14:191–202. https://doi.org/10.1007/s10495-008-0290-x.

[126] Raghuvar Gopal D V., Narkar AA, Badrinath Y, Mishra KP, Joshi DS. Protection of Ewing's sarcoma family tumor (ESFT) cell line SK-N-MC from betulinic acid induced apoptosis by α-DL-tocopherol. Toxicol Lett 2004;153:201–12. https://doi.org/10.1016/j.toxlet.2004.03.027.

[127] Tiwari R, Puthli A, Balakrishnan S, Sapra BK, Mishra KP. Betulinic acid-induced cytotoxicity in human breast tumor cell lines MCF-7 and T47D and its modification by tocopherol. Cancer Invest 2014;32:402–8. https://doi.org/10.3109/07357907.2014.933234.

[128] Tan YM, Yu R, Pezzuto JM. Betulinic acid-induced programmed cell death in human melanoma cells involves mitogen-activated protein kinase activation. Clin Cancer Res 2003;9:2866–75.

[129] Dillon LW, Pierce LCT, Lehman CE, Nikiforov YE, Wang YH. DNA topoisomerases participate in fragility of the oncogene RET. PLoS One 2013;8:1–15. https://doi.org/10.1371/journal.pone.0075741.

[130] Ganguly A, Das B, Roy A, Sen N, Dasgupta SB, Mukhopadhayay S, et al. Betulinic acid, a catalytic inhibitor of topoisomerase I, inhibits reactive oxygen species-mediated apoptotic topoisomerase I-DNA cleavable complex formation in prostate cancer cells but does not affect the process of cell death. Cancer Res 2007;67:11848–58. https://doi.org/10.1158/0008-5472.CAN-07-1615.

[131] Chowdhury RA, Mandal S, Mittra B, Sharma S, Mukhopadhyay S, Majumder HK. Betulinic acid, a potent inhibitor of eukaryotic topoisomerase I: identification of the inhibitory step, the major functional group responsible and development of more potent derivatives. Med Sci Monit 2002;8:254–60.

[132] Melzig MF, Bormann H. Betulinic acid inhibits aminopeptidase N activity. Planta Med 1998;64:655–7. https://doi.org/10.1055/s-2006-957542.

[133] Karna E, Szoka L, Palka JA. Betulinic acid inhibits the expression of hypoxia-inducible factor 1α and vascular endothelial growth factor in human endometrial adenocarcinoma cells. Mol Cell Biochem 2010;340:15–20. https://doi.org/10.1007/s11010-010-0395-8.

[134] Ren W, Qin L, Xu Y, Cheng N. Inhibition of betulinic acid to growth and angiogenesis of human colorectal cancer cell in nude mice. Chinese-German J Clin Oncol 2010;9:153–7. https://doi.org/10.1007/s10330-010-0002-1.

[135] Kwon HJ, Shim JS, Kim JH, Cho HY, Yum YN, Kim SH, et al. Betulinic acid inhibits growth factor-induced in vitro angiogenesis via the modulation of mitochondrial function in endothelial cells. Japanese J Cancer Res 2002;93:417–25. https://doi.org/10.1111/j.1349-7006.2002.tb01273.x.

[136] Dehelean CA, Feflea S, Ganta S, Amiji M. Anti-angiogenic effects of betulinic acid administered in nanoemulsion formulation using chorioallantoic membrane assay. J Biomed Nanotechnol 2011;7:317–24. https://doi.org/10.1166/jbn.2011.1297.

[137] Willmann M, Wacheck V, Buckley J, Nagy K, Thalhammer J, Paschke R, et al. Characterization of NVX-207, a novel betulinic acid-derived anti-cancer compound. Eur J Clin Invest 2009;39:384–94. https://doi.org/10.1111/j.1365-2362.2009.02105.x.

[138] Bache M, Bernhardt S, Passin S, Wichmann H, Hein A, Zschornak M, et al. Betulinic acid derivatives NVX-207 and B10 for treatment of glioblastoma—an in vitro study of cytotoxicity and radiosensitization. Int J Mol Sci 2014;15:19777–90. https://doi.org/10.3390/ijms151119777.

[139] Novelix Pharmaceuticals IJB. Compositions and methods using betulinic acid derivative NVX-207 and related compounds for treatment of inflammation and hyperkeratotic lesions. WO2009155070A2, 2009.

[140] Winum JY, Pastorekova S, Jakubickova L, Montero JL, Scozzafava A, Pastorek J, et al. Carbonic anhydrase inhibitors: Synthesis and inhibition of cytosolic/tumor-associated carbonic anhydrase isozymes I, II, and IX with bis-sulfamates. Bioorganic Med Chem Lett 2005;15:579–84. https://doi.org/10.1016/j.bmcl.2004.11.058.

[141] Federici C, Lugini L, Marino ML, Carta F, Iessi E, Azzarito T, et al. Lansoprazole and carbonic anhydrase IX inhibitors sinergize against human melanoma cells. J Enzyme Inhib Med Chem 2016;31:119–25. https://doi.org/10.1080/14756366.2016.1177525.

[142] Pastorekova S, Gillies RJ. The role of carbonic anhydrase IX in cancer development: links to hypoxia, acidosis, and beyond. Cancer Metastasis Rev 2019;38:65–77. https://doi.org/10.1007/s10555-019-09799-0.

[143] Supuran CT. Carbonic anhydrase inhibitors as emerging agents for the treatment and imaging of hypoxic tumors. Expert Opin Investig Drugs 2018;27:963–70. https://doi.org/10.1080/13543784.2018.1548608.

[144] Nogueira SAF, Torres SMF, Malone ED, Diaz SF, Jessen C, Gilbert S. Efficacy of imiquimod 5% cream in the treatment of equine sarcoids: A pilot study. Vet Dermatol 2006;17:259–65. https://doi.org/10.1111/j.1365-3164.2006.00526.x.

[145] Sloot S, Rashid OM, Sarnaik AA, Zager JS. Developments in intralesional therapy for metastatic melanoma. Cancer Control 2016;23:12–20. https://doi.org/10.1177/107327481602300104.

[146] Wang XJ, Chen JY, Fu LQ, Yan MJ. Recent advances in natural therapeutic approaches for the treatment of cancer. J Chemother 2020;32:53–65. https://doi.org/10.1080/1120009X.2019.1707417.

[147] Newman DJ, Cragg GM, Snader KM. Natural products as sources of new drugs over the period 1981-2002. J Nat Prod 2003;66:1022–37. https://doi.org/10.1021/np030096l.

[148] Amiri S, Dastghaib S, Ahmadi M, Mehrbod P, Khadem F, Behrouj H, et al. Betulin and its derivatives as novel compounds with different pharmacological effects. Biotechnol Adv 2020;38:1–39. https://doi.org/10.1016/j.biotechadv.2019.06.008.

[149] Ali-Seyed M, Jantan I, Vijayaraghavan K, Bukhari SNA. Betulinic Acid: Recent Advances in Chemical Modifications, Effective Delivery, and Molecular Mechanisms of a Promising Anticancer Therapy. Chem Biol Drug Des 2016;87:517–36. https://doi.org/10.1111/cbdd.12682.

[150] Selzer E, Pimentel E, Wacheck V, Schlegel W, Pehamberger H, Jansen B, et al. Effects of betulinic acid alone and in combination with irradiation in human melanoma cells. J Invest Dermatol 2000;114:935–40. https://doi.org/10.1046/j.1523-1747.2000.00972.x.

[151] Vanchanagiri K. Investigation of Novel Antitumor agents for New Approaches in Cancer Therapy. Martin-Luther-University Halle-Wittenberg, 2017.

[152] Scudiero D, McMahon J, Vistica D, Storeng R, Skehan P, Warren JT, et al. New Colorimetric Cytotoxicity Assay for Anticancer-Drug Screening. JNCI J Natl Cancer Inst 2007;82:1107–12. https://doi.org/10.1093/jnci/82.13.1107.

[153] Mosmann T. Rapid colorimetric assay for cellular growth and survival: application to proliferation and cytotoxicity assays. J ImmunolMethods 1983;65:55–63.

[154] Galgon T, Wohlrab W, Dräger B. Betulinic acid induces apoptosis in skin cancer cells and differentiation in normal human keratinocytes. Exp Dermatol 2005;14:736–43. https://doi.org/10.1111/j.1600-0625.2005.00352.x.

[155] Kessler JH, Mullauer FB, de Roo GM, Medema JP. Broad in vitro efficacy of plant-derived betulinic acid against cell lines derived from the most prevalent human cancer types. Cancer Lett 2007;251:132–45. https://doi.org/10.1016/j.canlet.2006.11.003.

[156] Surowiak P, Drag M, Materna V, Dietel M, Lage H. Betulinic acid exhibits stronger cytotoxic activity on the normal melanocyte NHEM-neo cell line than on drug-resistant and drug-sensitive MeWo melanoma cell lines. Mol Med Rep 2009;2:543–8. https://doi.org/10.3892/mmr_00000134.

[157] Sandberg F, Dutschewska H, Christov V, Spassov S. Spondianthus preussii var. glaber Engler. Pharmacological screening and occurrence of triterpenes. Acta Pharm Suec 1987;24:253–6.

[158] Mullauer FB, Van Bloois L, Daalhuisen JB, Ten Brink MS, Storm G, Medema JP, et al. Betulinic acid delivered in liposomes reduces growth of human lung and colon cancers in mice without causing systemic toxicity. Anticancer Drugs 2011;22:223–33. https://doi.org/10.1097/CAD.0b013e3283421035.

[159] Monteiro-Riviere NA, Bristol DG, Manning TO, Rogers RA, Riviere JE. Interspecies and Interregional Analysis of the Comparative Histologic Thickness and Laser Doppler Blood Flow Measurements at Five Cutaneous Sites in Nine Species. J Invest Dermatol 1990;95:582–6. https://doi.org/10.1111/1523-1747.ep12505567.

[160] Abd E, Yousef SA, Pastore MN, Telaprolu K, Mohammed YH, Namjoshi S, et al. Skin models for the testing of transdermal drugs. Clin Pharmacol Adv Appl 2016;8:163–76. https://doi.org/10.2147/CPAA.S64788.

[161] Mills PC, Cross SE. The effects of equine skin preparation on transdermal drug penetration in vitro. Can J Vet Res 2006;70:317–20.

[162] Stahl J, Niedorf F, Kietzmann M. The correlation between epidermal lipid composition and morphologic skin characteristics with percutaneous permeation: An interspecies comparison of substances with different lipophilicity. J Vet Pharmacol Ther 2011;34:502–7. https://doi.org/10.1111/j.1365-2885.2010.01246.x.

[163] Mills PC, Cross SE. Regional differences in the in vitro penetration of hydrocortisone through equine skin. J Vet Pharmacol Ther 2006;29:25–30. https://doi.org/10.1016/j.rvsc.2006.07.015.

[164] Wong D, Buechner-Maxwell V, Manning T. Equine Skin: Structure, Immunologic Function, and Methods of Diagnosing Disease. Compend Contin Educ Vet Am Ed 2005;27:463–73.

[165] Chang SK, Riviere JE. Effect of humidity and occlusion on the percutaneous absorption of parathion in vitro. Pharm Res 1993;10:152–5. https://doi.org/10.1023/A:1018901903243.

[166] Yao M, Gu C, Doyle FJ, Zhu H, Redmond RW, Kochevar IE. Why is rose Bengal more phototoxic to fibroblasts in vitro than in vivo? Photochem Photobiol 2014;90:297–305. https://doi.org/10.1111/php.12215.

[167] Sun T, Jackson S, Haycock JW, MacNeil S. Culture of skin cells in 3D rather than 2D improves their ability to survive exposure to cytotoxic agents. J Biotechnol 2006;122:372–81. https://doi.org/10.1016/j.jbiotec.2005.12.021.

[168] Pedersen JA, Swartz MA. Mechanobiology in the third dimension. Ann Biomed Eng 2005;33:1469–90. https://doi.org/10.1007/s10439-005-8159-4.

[169] Johnson W. Final report of the amended safety assessment of Glyceryl Laurate, Glyceryl Laurate SE, Glyceryl Laurate/Oleate, Glyceryl Adipate, Glyceryl Alginate, Glyceryl Arachidate, Glyceryl Arachidonate, Glyceryl Behenate, Glyceryl Caprate, Glyceryl Caprylate, Glyc. Int J Toxicol 2004;23:55–94. https://doi.org/10.1080/10915810490499064.

[170] Johnson W, Bergfeld WF, Belsito D V., Hill RA, Klaassen CD, Liebler D, et al. Safety Assessment of 1,2-Glycols as Used in Cosmetics. Int J Toxicol 2012;31:147S–168S. https://doi.org/10.1177/1091581812460409.

[171] Johnson W. Final Report on the Safety Assessment of Cetearyl Alcohol, Cetyl Alcohol, Isostearyl Alcohol, Myristyl Alcohol, and Behenyl Alcohol. J Am Coll Toxicol 1988;7:395–413. https://doi.org/10.1080/10915810802550835.

[172] Kapałczyńska M, Kolenda T, Przybyła W, Zajączkowska M, Teresiak A, Filas V, et al. 2D and 3D cell cultures – a comparison of different types of cancer cell cultures. Arch Med Sci 2016;14:910–9. https://doi.org/10.5114/aoms.2016.63743.

[173] Ferreira D, Adega F, Chaves R. The Importance of Cancer Cell Lines as in vitro Models in Cancer Methylome Analysis and Anticancer Drugs Testing. Oncogenomics Cancer Proteomics - Nov. Approaches Biomarkers Discov. Ther. Targets Cancer, vol. 3, InTech; 2013, p. 139–66. https://doi.org/10.5772/53110.

[174] van Staveren WCG, Solís DYW, Hébrant A, Detours V, Dumont JE, Maenhaut C. Human cancer cell lines: Experimental models for cancer cells in situ? For cancer stem cells? Biochim Biophys Acta - Rev Cancer 2009;1795:92–103. https://doi.org/10.1016/j.bbcan.2008.12.004.

[175] Witz IP. Yin-Yang activities and vicious cycles in the tumor microenvironment. Cancer Res 2008;68:9–13. https://doi.org/10.1158/0008-5472.CAN-07-2917.

[176] Tokudome Y, Katayanagi M, Hashimoto F. Esterase activity and intracellular localization in reconstructed human epidermal cultured skin models. Ann Dermatol 2015;27:269–74. https://doi.org/10.5021/ad.2015.27.3.269.

[177] Jha SK, Dey S, Karki R. Microemulsions- Potential Carrier for Improved Drug Delivery. Asian J Biomed Pharm Sci 2011;1:5–9.

[178] Wachsberger PR, Burd R, Wahl ML, Leeper DB. Betulinic acid sensitization of low pH adapted human melanoma cells to hyperthermia. Int J Hyperth 2002;18:153–64. https://doi.org/10.1080/02656730110091333.

[179] Noda Y, Kaiya T, Kohda K, Kawazoe Y. Enhanced Cytotoxicity of Some Triterpenes toward Leukemia L1210 Cells Cultured in Low pH Media: Possibility of a New Mode of Cell Killing. Chem Pharm Bull (Tokyo) 1997;45:1665–70. https://doi.org/10.1248/cpb.45.1665.

[180] Vaupel P, Kallinowski F, Okunieff P. Blood Flow, Oxygen and Nutrient Supply, and Metabolic Microenvironment of Human Tumors: A Review. Cancer Res 1989;49:6449–65.

[181] Boussadia Z, Lamberti J, Mattei F, Pizzi E, Puglisi R, Zanetti C, et al. Acidic microenvironment plays a key role in human melanoma progression through a sustained exosome mediated transfer of clinically relevant metastatic molecules. J Exp Clin Cancer Res 2018;37:1–15. https://doi.org/10.1186/s13046-018-0915-z.

[182] Jain RK, Martin JD, Stylianopoulos T. The Role of Mechanical Forces in Tumor Growth and Therapy. Annu Rev Biomed Eng 2014;16:321–46. https://doi.org/10.1146/annurev-bioeng-071813-105259.

[183] Azimi F, Scolyer RA, Rumcheva P, Moncrieff M, Murali R, McCarthy SW, et al. Tumor-infiltrating lymphocyte grade is an independent predictor of sentinel lymph node status and survival in patients with cutaneous melanoma. J Clin Oncol 2012;30:2678–83. https://doi.org/10.1200/JCO.2011.37.8539.

[184] Fu Q, Chen N, Ge C, Li R, Li Z, Zeng B, et al. Prognostic value of tumor-infiltrating lymphocytes in melanoma: a systematic review and meta-analysis. Oncoimmunology 2019;8:1–14. https://doi.org/10.1080/2162402X.2019.1593806.

[185] Moser K, Kriwet K, Naik A, Kalia YN, Guy RH. Passive skin penetration enhancement and its quantification in vitro. Eur J Pharm Biopharm 2001;52:103–12. https://doi.org/10.1016/S0939-6411(01)00166-7.

[186] Lopes LB. Overcoming the cutaneous barrier with microemulsions. Pharmaceutics 2014;6:52–77. https://doi.org/10.3390/pharmaceutics6010052.

[187] Rastrelli M, Tropea S, Rossi CR, Alaibac M. Melanoma: epidemiology, risk factors, pathogenesis, diagnosis and classification. In Vivo (Brooklyn) 2014;28:1005–11. https://doi.org/10.32388/7XJ0GW.

[188] van der Weyden L, Patton EE, Wood GA, Foote AK, Brenn T, Arends MJ, et al. Cross-species models of human melanoma. J Pathol 2016;238:152–65. https://doi.org/10.1002/path.4632.

[189] Lichtenstein F, Iqbal A, de Lima Will SEA, Bosch RV, DeOcesano-Pereira C, Goldfeder MB, et al. Modulation of stress and immune response by Amblyomin-X results in tumor cell death in a horse melanoma model. Sci Reports Nat Res 2020;10:1–15. https://doi.org/10.1038/s41598-020-63275-2.

[190] Fulda S, Jeremias I, Debatin KM. Cooperation of betulinic acid and TRAIL to induce apoptosis in tumor cells. Oncogene 2004;23:7611–20. https://doi.org/10.1038/sj.onc.1207970.

[191] Fulda S. Betulinic acid for cancer treatment and prevention. Int J Mol Sci 2008;9:1096–107. https://doi.org/10.3390/ijms9061096.

[192] National Institute of Biomedical Imaging and Bioengineering. Drug Delivery Systems - Getting Drugs to Their Targets in a Controlled Manner. Natl Inst Biomed Imaging Bioeng 2013.

[193] Notman R, Den Otter WK, Noro MG, Briels WJ, Anwar J. The permeability enhancing mechanism of DMSO in ceramide bilayers simulated by molecular dynamics. Biophys J 2007;93:2056–68. https://doi.org/10.1529/biophysj.107.104703.

[194] Naik A, Pechtold LARM, Potts RO, Guy RH. Mechanism of oleic acid-induced skin penetration enhancement in vivo in humans. J Control Release 1995;37:299–306. https://doi.org/10.1016/0168-3659(95)00088-7.

[195] Hadgraft J. Passive enhancement strategies in topical and transdermal drug delivery. Int J Pharm 1999;184:1–6. https://doi.org/10.1016/S0378-5173(99)00095-2.

[196] Cristina F, Vieira L, Badra Bentley MVL. Confocal Laser Scanning Microscopy as a Tool for the Investigation of Skin Drug Delivery Systems and Diagnosis of Skin Disorders. Confocal Laser Microsc. - Princ. Appl. Med. Biol. Food Sci., vol. i, InTech; 2013, p. 99–140. https://doi.org/10.5772/55995.

Affidavit

I herewith declare that I autonomously carried out the PhD thesis entitled:

"*In vitro* and *in vivo* development of a topical drug for the treatment of equine skin cancer – based on naturally occurring and synthetically modified substances in plane bark"

No third party assistance has been used.

I did not receive any assistance in return for payment by consulting agencies or any other person. No one received any kind of payment for direct or indirect assistance in correlation to the content of the submitted thesis.

I conducted the project at the following institutions:

- Clinic for Horses, University of Veterinary Medicine Hannover, Foundation
- Department of Pharmacology, Toxicology and Pharmacy, University of Veterinary Medicine Hannover, Foundation
- Lipizzaner Stud Piber – Spanish Riding School Vienna (Austria)

The thesis has not been submitted elsewhere for an exam, as thesis or for evaluation in a similar context.

I hereby affirm the above statements to be complete and true to the best of my knowledge.

Lisa A. Weber

Acknowledgements

During the last three years I have learned a lot and was able to develop myself for which I am very grateful. Many people have accompanied me during my PhD research and I would like to take the opportunity to thank them.

First, I would like to express my sincere gratitude to my supervisors Prof. Dr. Jessika-M.V. Cavalleri, Prof. Dr. Karsten Feige, and Prof. Dr. Manfred Kietzmann for excellent professional and mental support during the last three years. In particular I would like to thank Prof. Dr. Jessika-M.V. Cavalleri for giving me the opportunity to work on this project, for continuous and encouraging support during the experimental and writing processes and the willingness to advise me in all PhD- and career-related questions at any time. I would like to express my profound thanks to Prof. Dr. Karsten Feige for well thought-out and sound suggestions to solve problems that have arisen, taking time for honest and constructive advice before presentations at national and international congresses, and helpful guidance in career questions. Prof. Dr. Manfred Kietzmann's inspiring and excellent ideas contributed enormously to the progress of the project and through his humorous and positive way he supported me especially when the "doctoral student's mood curve" showed a downward trend.
I am sincerely grateful for that.

I also owe a debt of gratitude to Dr. Jessica Meißner, who shared her knowledge about cell culture experiments, Franz-type diffusion cell studies and data analysis with me and who did a lot of proofreading. Especially at the beginning of the project, she answered my many questions in such a patient and good-humoured way that after each conversation I was even more motivated to continue working.

Furthermore, I am indebted to our collaboration partners from the Biozentrum of the Martin-Luther-University Halle-Wittenberg, Biosolutions Halle GmbH and Skinomics GmbH for a harmoniously collaboration. "The essence of collaborative partnerships is for all parties to mutually benefit from working together", Wikipedia says. Reflecting the last three years, I would say: we definitely did.
A special thanks to Prof. Dr. Reinhard Paschke (Biozentrum) for project conceptualization and providing his excellent expertise whenever needed. Furthermore, I would like to thank Anne Funtan (Biozentrum) for answering my many questions regarding chemical issues, introducing me to FACS analysis, discussing cell culture results, her valuable contributions especially to manuscript II, and becoming a friend during the project.

I would like to express my gratitude to Dr. Jutta Kalbitz (Biosolutions Halle GmbH) who did an incredible job in the last three years. She analyzed more samples for the ZIM project and the current PhD work by HPLC than I can express my gratitude in words. I really appreciated her fast and reliable way of working and the interesting and constructive discussions we had. Furthermore, I am happy to acknowledge Dr. Julia Michael, Dr. Konstanze Bosse and Christian Sporn (all Skinomics GmbH) for providing test formulations and for constructive discussions and competent advice during the project meetings. Sara Bodamer and Linus Gohlke have also made valuable contributions to the pharmaceutical development of the test formulations.

I would like to thank Dr. Barbara Pratscher (Division of Small Animal Internal Medicine, Department for Companion Animals and Horses, University of Veterinary Medicine Vienna, Austria) and Dr. Sabine Brandt (Research Group Oncology, University of Veterinary Medicine Vienna) for providing equine malignant melanoma cells eRGO1 and equine sarcoid cells sRGO1 and sRGO2 and the opportunity of conducting cell culture experiments (melanoma cell characterization) in their laboratory. In particular I would like to thank Dr. Barbara Pratscher for valuable and inspiring discussions about cell culture methods and results as well as the pathophysiology of equine malignant melanoma.

I am grateful to Carolin Groß who taught me the practical work in the cell culture lab and who always helped me with all kinds of laboratory questions. I further thank my colleagues at the Department for Pharmacology, Toxicology and Pharmacy for a nice time together at the institute with emphasis on the “Salattag”.

I wish to thank the PhD-Commission of the Hannover Graduate School for Veterinary Pathobiology, Neuroinfectiology, and Translational Medicine (particularly Prof. Dr. Beatrice Grummer, Dr. Tina Selle, and Tanja Czeslik) for their constant help, organization, and financial support.

Further, I would like to thank the Spanish riding school Vienna (Austria) for the opportunity to perform the efficacy study at the Lipizzaner Stud Piber. The great team of the stud and those beautiful horses have definitely contributed positively to the fact that my PhD time will remain unforgettable.

I would like to express my greatest thanks to Julien Delarocque, who has not only been an incredibly helpful PhD colleague from day 1, but also a loyal friend. Thank you for all the valuable discussions in which you immersed yourself into specific questions of my project, thank you for your help with statistical issues, thank you for your motivating words when I doubted. I have learned a lot from you.

Florian Frers completes the "PhD crew JFL". Thank you for good and funny times in private life, in the clinic and at congresses, for supporting conversations, and your friendship. Further thanks and greetings go to the whole team of the Clinic for Horses.

Thanks to Daphna Emanuel and my fellow PhD students Mona Hassan, Sebastian Meller, PhD, Maren Schenke, PhD, and Sarah Schwarz for giving me a good time in Hannover. Prof. Dr. Katharina Krämer proofread many parts of the thesis and did a great job on it.

I would like to thank my flat mate and PhD mate Selma Staege, with whom I could share all good and less pleasant experiences in professional and private matters and who became a friend for life. I am genuinely thankful for your support and heartiness.

Thank you so much, Nikolas Krämer, for your unique and contagious positive energy, your constant support and believing in me at any time.

Finally, my sincerest and most heartfelt gratitude is dedicated to my family, especially to my parents Ute and Rudi Weber. Throughout life, you have always been greatly supportive and encouraging. I am exceptionally thankful for your reliance, your love, and your never-ending help.

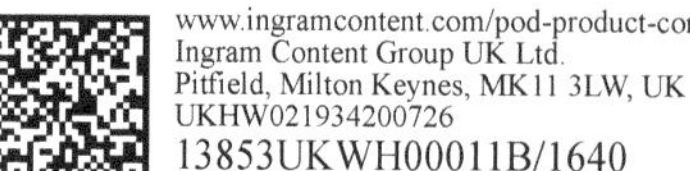
www.ingramcontent.com/pod-product-compliance
Ingram Content Group UK Ltd.
Pitfield, Milton Keynes, MK11 3LW, UK
UKHW021934200726
13853UKWH00011B/1640